CKD STAGE 3 COOKBOOK FOR SENIORS

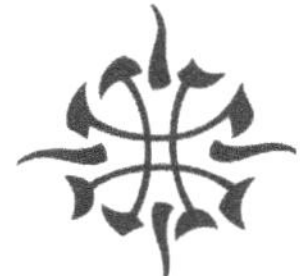

Simple and Flavorful Meals that there recipes are Low in Sodium, Potassium, and Phosphorus Recipes/ 30-Days Meal Plan

Dr Jose B. Willis

Chapter 1:

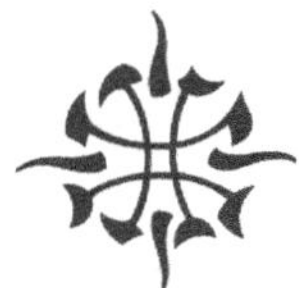

INTRODUCTION

Living with CKD can present unique challenges, and it's crucial to understand the importance of a kidney-friendly diet. Stage 3 CKD indicates moderate kidney damage, and it becomes increasingly vital to manage your diet to support kidney function and overall health. With the right approach, you can still enjoy a wide variety of flavorful and satisfying meals while taking care of your kidneys.

In this cookbook, we will delve into the dietary guidelines for CKD Stage 3, highlighting the key nutrients to limit or monitor and those that are beneficial for your well-being. You'll discover the importance of controlling sodium, potassium, and phosphorus intake, as well as understanding the role of protein, fluid balance, and other essential nutrients in managing CKD.

We understand that cooking for CKD Stage 3 can be overwhelming, especially if you're accustomed to certain ingredients and flavors. That's why this cookbook is here to guide you through the process, introducing you to kidney-friendly ingredients, cooking techniques, and flavor-enhancing herbs and spices that can make your meals both healthy and delicious.

Throughout this book, you'll find a diverse selection of recipes, carefully crafted to meet the nutritional needs of seniors with CKD Stage 3. From nourishing breakfast options to satisfying main courses and delightful desserts, we have included a range of recipes to suit various tastes and dietary preferences. Each recipe comes with detailed instructions, nutrition facts, and serving suggestions to make it easier for you to plan your meals and keep track of your nutrient intake.

Remember, this cookbook is not intended to replace the advice of your healthcare professional or registered dietitian. It is always important to consult with a healthcare professional to personalize your dietary plan according to your specific needs and medical condition.

We hope this CKD Stage 3 Cookbook for Seniors becomes a valuable resource in your journey towards managing your kidney health while enjoying delicious meals. Let's embark on this culinary adventure together and discover a world of flavors that will help you thrive on your CKD journey!

Understanding CKD Stage 3:

Chronic Kidney Disease (CKD) is a progressive condition characterized by the gradual loss of kidney function over time. CKD is classified into five stages, with Stage 3 indicating moderate kidney damage. It is crucial to have a good understanding of CKD Stage 3 in order to manage the condition effectively.

In Stage 3, the kidneys are still functioning, but not as efficiently as they should. This means they may have difficulty filtering waste products and excess fluids from the body. It's essential to monitor and manage your kidney health during this stage to prevent further damage and maintain overall well-being.

One of the primary goals in managing CKD Stage 3 is to slow down the progression of the disease and maintain kidney function for as long as possible. This can be achieved through lifestyle modifications, including adopting a kidney-friendly diet.

When it comes to CKD Stage 3, understanding your nutritional needs is paramount. A kidney-friendly diet aims to minimize the workload on the kidneys and maintain a balance of essential nutrients to support overall health. Let's delve into the key nutritional considerations for CKD patients:

1. Protein: Protein is an important nutrient for the body, but in CKD Stage 3, it is necessary to monitor protein intake. Consuming excessive protein can strain the kidneys. However, an adequate amount of high-quality protein is still essential for maintaining muscle mass and supporting overall health. Your healthcare professional or dietitian will guide you on the appropriate protein intake for your specific needs.

2. Sodium: Sodium, commonly found in salt, can contribute to fluid retention and high blood pressure, both of which can put additional strain on the kidneys. It is important to limit sodium in your diet by reducing the consumption of processed and packaged foods, as they often contain high amounts of sodium. Instead, opt for fresh ingredients and use herbs and spices to add flavor to your meals.

3. Potassium: In CKD Stage 3, the kidneys may have difficulty maintaining the proper balance of potassium in the body. High levels of potassium can be harmful, leading to irregular heartbeats and other complications. It is important to moderate potassium intake by avoiding high-potassium foods such as bananas, oranges, tomatoes, and potatoes. Your healthcare professional or dietitian will guide you on the appropriate potassium level for your specific needs.

4. Phosphorus: The kidneys play a crucial role in regulating phosphorus levels in the body. In CKD Stage 3, phosphorus can accumulate, leading to bone and heart problems. It is important to limit phosphorus-rich foods such as dairy products, nuts, and processed meats. Additionally, taking phosphate binders as prescribed by your healthcare professional can help control phosphorus levels.

5. Fluid Balance: Maintaining a proper fluid balance is essential for individuals with CKD Stage 3. Your healthcare professional or dietitian will guide you on the appropriate fluid intake based on your specific needs, considering factors such as urine output and the presence of other medical conditions.

In addition to these key considerations, it is important to focus on maintaining a balanced and varied diet that includes a range of fruits, vegetables, whole grains, and healthy fats. These provide essential vitamins, minerals, and antioxidants that support overall health and well-being.

Remember, each individual's nutritional needs may vary, and it's crucial to work closely with your healthcare professional or registered dietitian to develop a personalized dietary plan that suits your specific requirements. They will take into account your overall health, kidney function, and any other medical conditions you may have.

By understanding your nutritional needs and making informed food choices, you can take an active role in managing CKD Stage 3 and promoting your overall well-being. The following chapters of this cookbook will provide you with delicious recipes that align with the dietary considerations for CKD Stage 3, helping you create nourishing and kidney-friendly meals.

How to Use This Cookbook:

This cookbook is designed to be a practical guide for seniors living with CKD Stage 3 and their caregivers. Here are some tips on how to make the most out of this cookbook:

1. Familiarize Yourself with the Recipes: Take some time to browse through the recipes and get acquainted with the variety of dishes included. Note down the recipes that catch your interest and fit your dietary preferences.

2. Read the Recipe Instructions: Before starting any recipe, read through the instructions carefully. Familiarize yourself with the cooking techniques and equipment required. This will help you plan your time and ensure a smooth cooking process.

3. Note the Serving Sizes: Each recipe in this cookbook provides serving sizes and nutritional information. Pay attention to the serving sizes to ensure you're consuming appropriate portions that align with your dietary needs.

4. Adjust the Recipes: Feel free to adjust the recipes based on your taste preferences and dietary requirements. If you need to modify ingredient quantities or make substitutions, refer to the section on ingredient substitutions and modifications for guidance.

5. Plan Your Meals: Use this cookbook as a tool to plan your meals for the week. Take note of the recipes you want to try and create a shopping list accordingly. Planning ahead can help you stay organized and ensure you have all the necessary ingredients on hand.

6. Experiment and Customize: Don't be afraid to add your own personal touch to the recipes. Use herbs, spices, and seasonings to enhance flavors and make the dishes more enjoyable for your palate. Cooking should be a creative and enjoyable experience!

7. Keep Track of Nutrients: If you're closely monitoring your nutrient intake, you may want to keep a food diary or consult with a registered dietitian. This will help you track your sodium, potassium, phosphorus, and protein consumption, ensuring you stay within the recommended limits.

Tips for Cooking with CKD:

Cooking with CKD Stage 3 in mind requires some special considerations. Here are a few tips to keep in mind while preparing kidney-friendly meals:

1. Rinse Canned Foods: If you're using canned foods like beans or vegetables, rinse them thoroughly under running water to reduce the sodium content.

2. Soak High-Potassium Foods: If you're using high-potassium vegetables like potatoes or winter squash, consider soaking them in water for a few hours to help reduce their potassium content.

3. Opt for Fresh Ingredients: Whenever possible, choose fresh ingredients over processed or packaged foods. Fresh fruits, vegetables, and lean proteins are generally lower in sodium and other additives.

4. Use Herbs and Spices: To enhance the flavor of your meals without relying on salt, experiment with herbs and spices. Options like garlic, ginger, turmeric, rosemary, and basil can add depth and taste to your dishes.

5. Practice Portion Control: Pay attention to portion sizes to avoid overeating. Use measuring cups or a food scale to ensure you're consuming appropriate amounts of protein, grains, and other ingredients.

Ingredient Substitutions and Modifications:

Sometimes, you may need to make substitutions or modifications to the recipes to suit your dietary needs or ingredient availability. Here are a few common ingredient swaps you can consider:

1. Salt Substitutes: If you need to limit sodium, try using salt substitutes or herbs and spices to add flavor to your dishes.

2. Low-Potassium Substitutions: For high-potassium ingredients like bananas, tomatoes, or oranges, you can substitute with lower-potassium options such as apples, cucumbers, or berries.

3. Phosphorus Control: If you need to limit phosphorus, choose low-phosphorus dairy alternatives like almond milk, rice milk, or coconut milk instead of regular cow's milk.

4. Protein Modifications: If you need to adjust your protein intake, consult with your healthcare professional or dietitian for guidance on choosing appropriate protein sources and portion sizes.

Remember, it's important to consult with your healthcare professional or registered dietitian before making any significant modifications to your diet. They can provide personalized recommendations and ensure you're making appropriate choices for your specific needs.

By following the guidance in this cookbook, incorporating tips for cooking with CKD, and making necessary ingredient substitutions or modifications, you can confidently prepare kidney-friendly meals that are both delicious and supportive of your overall health. Enjoy your culinary journey.

CKD Stage 3 Meal Plan for Seniors

Always remember:

- Limit sodium intake to around 1,500mg per day.
- Monitor potassium and phosphorus intake as advised by your doctor.
- Choose whole grains over refined grains.
- Include plenty of fruits and vegetables (be mindful of potassium content in some).
- Use herbs and spices for flavor instead of salt.
- Drink plenty of water throughout the day (unless fluid restricted by your doctor).

Day 1:

- **Breakfast:** Scrambled eggs with chopped tomatoes and spinach, whole-wheat toast with avocado
- **Lunch:** Grilled chicken salad with mixed greens, low-sodium vinaigrette, apple slices
- **Dinner:** Baked salmon with roasted asparagus and brown rice

Day 2:

- **Breakfast:** Oatmeal with berries and a sprinkle of chopped nuts
- **Lunch:** Vegetarian lentil soup with whole-wheat bread, side salad
- **Dinner:** Turkey chili with low-sodium kidney beans and cornbread (made with a potassium-substitute)

Day 3:

- **Breakfast:** Whole-wheat pancakes with blueberries and low-fat yogurt
- **Lunch:** Tuna salad sandwich on whole-wheat bread with lettuce and tomato, side salad
- **Dinner:** Chicken stir-fry with brown rice noodles and mixed vegetables (low-potassium options recommended)

Day 4:

- **Breakfast:** Smoothie made with low-fat yogurt, banana, and spinach
- **Lunch:** Black bean burgers on whole-wheat buns with sweet potato fries
- **Dinner:** Baked cod with roasted Brussels sprouts and quinoa

Day 5:

- **Breakfast:** Poached eggs on whole-wheat toast with sliced avocado
- **Lunch:** Chicken Caesar salad with a light, low-sodium dressing

- **Dinner:** Vegetarian chili with chopped vegetables and brown rice

Day 6:

- **Breakfast:** Whole-wheat pancakes with applesauce and a sprinkle of cinnamon
- **Lunch:** Leftover chicken stir-fry from Day 3
- **Dinner:** Baked salmon with steamed broccoli and brown rice

Day 7:

- **Breakfast:** Scrambled eggs with chopped mushrooms and onions, whole-wheat toast
- **Lunch:** Chicken salad sandwich on whole-wheat bread with lettuce and tomato, carrot sticks
- **Dinner:** Vegetarian lasagna made with whole-wheat noodles and low-sodium ricotta cheese (watch potassium content in vegetables)

Day 8:

- **Breakfast:** Oatmeal with chopped nuts and a drizzle of honey
- **Lunch:** Tuna noodle casserole made with whole-wheat pasta and low-sodium cream of mushroom soup
- **Dinner:** Turkey meatballs with marinara sauce and whole-wheat spaghetti

Day 9:

- **Breakfast:** Whole-wheat waffles with banana slices and low-fat yogurt
- **Lunch:** Leftover vegetarian chili from Day 5
- **Dinner:** Baked chicken breast with roasted sweet potato and green beans

Day 10:

- **Breakfast:** Smoothie made with low-fat yogurt, berries, and spinach
- **Lunch:** Chicken salad with mixed greens, low-sodium vinaigrette, pear slices
- **Dinner:** Baked fish with roasted cauliflower and quinoa

Day 11:

- **Breakfast:** Whole-wheat pancakes with ricotta cheese and peaches
- **Lunch:** Lentil soup with a side salad and whole-wheat crackers
- **Dinner:** Baked cod with roasted zucchini and quinoa

Day 12:

- **Breakfast:** Scrambled eggs with chopped bell peppers and onions, whole-wheat toast
- **Lunch:** Chicken Caesar salad with a light, low-sodium dressing and whole-wheat croutons (watch potassium in dressing)
- **Dinner:** Vegetarian chili with brown rice and a dollop of low-fat sour cream (avoid high-potassium options)

Day 13:

- **Breakfast:** Oatmeal with chopped pear and a sprinkle of cinnamon
- **Lunch:** Turkey and vegetable wrap on a whole-wheat tortilla with hummus
- **Dinner:** Baked salmon with steamed asparagus and brown rice

Day 14:

- **Breakfast:** Smoothie made with low-fat yogurt, banana, and spinach

- **Lunch:** Leftover vegetarian chili from Day 11
- **Dinner:** Chicken stir-fry with brown rice and low-potassium vegetables (broccoli, carrots)

Day 15:

- **Breakfast:** Poached eggs on whole-wheat toast with sliced avocado
- **Lunch:** Tuna salad sandwich on whole-wheat bread with lettuce and tomato, side salad
- **Dinner:** Vegetarian lasagna with whole-wheat noodles and low-sodium ricotta cheese (watch potassium content in vegetables)

Day 16:

- **Breakfast:** Whole-wheat pancakes with applesauce and a sprinkle of cinnamon
- **Lunch:** Leftover chicken stir-fry from Day 14
- **Dinner:** Baked cod with roasted Brussels sprouts and quinoa

Day 17:

- **Breakfast:** Scrambled eggs with chopped mushrooms and spinach, whole-wheat toast
- **Lunch:** Chicken noodle soup with whole-wheat noodles (low-sodium broth) and a side salad
- **Dinner:** Turkey meatballs with marinara sauce and whole-wheat spaghetti

Day 18:

- **Breakfast:** Oatmeal with chopped nuts and a drizzle of honey
- **Lunch:** Tuna melt on whole-wheat bread with low-sodium cheese (watch potassium content)

- **Dinner:** Baked chicken breast with roasted sweet potato and green beans

Day 19:

- **Breakfast:** Smoothie made with low-fat yogurt, berries, and spinach
- **Lunch:** Chicken salad with mixed greens, low-sodium vinaigrette, pear slices
- **Dinner:** Baked fish with roasted cauliflower and quinoa

Day 20:

- **Breakfast:** Whole-wheat waffles with banana slices and low-fat yogurt
- **Lunch:** Lentil soup with a side salad and whole-wheat crackers
- **Dinner:** Vegetarian chili with brown rice and a sprinkle of grated Parmesan cheese (avoid high-potassium options)

Day 21:

- **Breakfast:** Whole-wheat muffins with blueberries and a sprinkle of chopped nuts
- **Lunch:** Chicken Caesar salad with a light, low-sodium dressing and whole-wheat croutons (watch potassium in dressing)
- **Dinner:** Baked salmon with roasted asparagus and quinoa

Day 22:

- **Breakfast:** Scrambled eggs with chopped tomatoes and spinach, whole-wheat toast
- **Lunch:** Turkey and vegetable wrap on a whole-wheat tortilla with hummus
- **Dinner:** Vegetarian chili with brown rice and a dollop of low-fat sour cream (avoid high-potassium options)

Day 23:

- **Breakfast:** Oatmeal with chopped apple and a sprinkle of cinnamon
- **Lunch:** Tuna salad sandwich on whole-wheat bread with lettuce and tomato, side salad
- **Dinner:** Chicken stir-fry with brown rice noodles and low-potassium vegetables (broccoli, carrots)

Day 24:

- **Breakfast:** Smoothie made with low-fat yogurt, banana, and spinach
- **Lunch:** Leftover vegetarian chili from Day 22
- **Dinner:** Baked cod with roasted Brussels sprouts and quinoa

Day 25:

- **Breakfast:** Poached eggs on whole-wheat toast with sliced avocado
- **Lunch:** Chicken noodle soup with whole-wheat noodles (low-sodium broth) and a side salad
- **Dinner:** Turkey meatballs with marinara sauce and whole-wheat spaghetti

Day 26:

- **Breakfast:** Whole-wheat pancakes with ricotta cheese and peaches
- **Lunch:** Leftover chicken stir-fry from Day 23
- **Dinner:** Baked chicken breast with roasted sweet potato and green beans

Day 27:

- **Breakfast:** Scrambled eggs with chopped mushrooms and onions, whole-wheat toast
- **Lunch:** Lentil soup with a side salad and whole-wheat crackers
- **Dinner:** Vegetarian lasagna with whole-wheat noodles and low-sodium ricotta cheese (watch potassium content in vegetables)

Day 28:

- **Breakfast:** Oatmeal with chopped nuts and a drizzle of honey
- **Lunch:** Tuna melt on whole-wheat bread with low-sodium cheese (watch potassium content)
- **Dinner:** Baked fish with roasted cauliflower and quinoa

Day 29:

- **Breakfast:** Smoothie made with low-fat yogurt, berries, and spinach
- **Lunch:** Chicken salad with mixed greens, low-sodium vinaigrette, pear slices
- **Dinner:** Vegetarian chili with brown rice and a sprinkle of grated Parmesan cheese (avoid high-potassium options)

Day 30:

- **Breakfast:** Whole-wheat waffles with banana slices and low-fat yogurt
- **Lunch:** Scrambled eggs with chopped bell peppers and onions, whole-wheat toast
- **Dinner:** Baked salmon with steamed asparagus and brown rice

Enjoy these scrumptious doses of delicious and nutritious meals designed to support your CKD management!

Chapter 2:

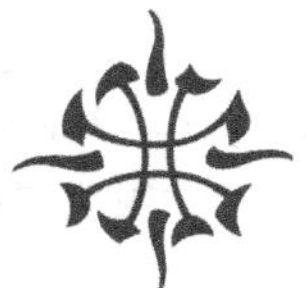

Oatmeal with Fresh Berries:

Preparation Time: 5 minutes

Cooking Time: 10 minutes

Servings: 2

Ingredients:

- 1 cup rolled oats

- 2 cups water

- Pinch of salt

- 1/2 cup fresh berries (such as blueberries, strawberries, or raspberries)

- 1 tablespoon chopped nuts (optional)

- 1 tablespoon honey or a low-sugar sweetener (optional)

Directions:

1. In a saucepan, bring water to a boil.

2. Add the rolled oats and a pinch of salt. Reduce the heat to low and simmer for 5-7 minutes, stirring occasionally, until the oats are cooked and have reached your desired consistency.

3. Remove the oatmeal from the heat and divide it into two bowls.

4. Top each bowl with fresh berries and chopped nuts, if desired.

5. Drizzle with honey or a low-sugar sweetener, if desired.

6. Serve warm and enjoy!

Nutrition (per serving):

- Calories: 200

- Protein: 6g

- Carbohydrates: 36g

- Fat: 4g

- Fiber: 5g

Scrambled Egg Whites with Spinach:

Preparation Time: 5 minutes

Cooking Time: 10 minutes

Servings: 2

Ingredients:

- 4 large egg whites

- 1 cup fresh spinach leaves

- 1 tablespoon olive oil

- Salt and pepper to taste

Directions:

1. In a medium bowl, whisk the egg whites until frothy. Season with salt and pepper.

2. Heat olive oil in a non-stick skillet over medium heat.

3. Add the spinach leaves and sauté for 1-2 minutes until wilted.

4. Pour the whisked egg whites into the skillet with the spinach.

5. Cook, stirring gently, until the eggs are cooked through and scrambled to your desired consistency.

6. Remove from heat and serve hot.

Nutrition (per serving):

- Calories: 80

- Protein: 14g

- Carbohydrates: 1g

- Fat: 2g

- Fiber: 0g

Low-Phosphorus Smoothie:

Preparation Time: 5 minutes

Servings: 1

Ingredients:

- 1 cup unsweetened almond milk

- 1/2 cup frozen berries (such as strawberries, blueberries, or raspberries)

- 1/2 small banana

- 1 tablespoon almond butter

- Ice cubes (optional)

Directions:

1. In a blender, combine almond milk, frozen berries, banana, and almond butter.

2. Blend until smooth and creamy.

3. If desired, add a few ice cubes and blend again until well combined and chilled.

4. Pour into a glass and enjoy!

Nutrition (per serving):

- Calories: 250

- Protein: 6g

- Carbohydrates: 28g

- Fat: 15g

- Fiber: 7g

Apple Cinnamon Muffins:

Preparation Time: 15 minutes

Cooking Time: 25 minutes

Servings: 12 muffins

Ingredients:

- 2 cups all-purpose flour

- 1 teaspoon baking powder

- 1/2 teaspoon baking soda

- 1/2 teaspoon ground cinnamon

- 1/4 teaspoon salt

- 2 large eggs

- 1/2 cup unsweetened applesauce

- 1/2 cup low-fat plain yogurt

- 1/4 cup honey or a low-sugar sweetener

- 1 teaspoon vanilla extract

- 1 medium apple, peeled and diced

Directions:

1. Preheat the oven to 350°F (175°C). Line a muffin tin with paper liners or lightly grease the cups.

2. In a large bowl, whisk together the flour, baking powder, baking soda, cinnamon, and salt.

3. In another bowl, beat the eggs, applesauce, yogurt, honey, and vanilla extract until well combined.

4. Pour the wet ingredients into the dry ingredients and stir until just combined. Do not overmix.

5. Gently fold in the diced apple.

6. Divide the batter evenly among the muffin cups, filling each about 3/4 full.

7. Bake for 20-25 minutes or until a toothpick inserted into the center of a muffin comes out clean.

8. Remove from the oven and let cool in the pan for a few minutes before transferring to a wire rack to cool completely.

Nutrition (per muffin):

- Calories: 130

- Protein: 3g

- Carbohydrates: 27g

- Fat: 1g

- Fiber: 1g

Rice Porridge with Almond Milk:

Preparation Time: 5 minutes

Cooking Time: 30 minutes

Servings: 2

Ingredients:

- 1/2 cup white rice

- 2 cups unsweetened almond milk

- 1 tablespoon honey or a low-sugar sweetener

- 1/4 teaspoon ground cinnamon

- 1/4 teaspoon vanilla extract

- Sliced almonds for garnish (optional)

Directions:

1. Rinse the rice under cold water until the water runs clear.

2. In a saucepan, combine the rinsed rice and almond milk. Bring to a boil over medium heat.

3. Reduce the heat to low, cover the saucepan, and simmer for about 25-30 minutes, stirring occasionally, until the rice is cooked and the mixture has thickened to a porridge consistency.

4. Stir in the honey, ground cinnamon, and vanilla extract.

5. Remove from heat and let it cool slightly.

6. Serve the rice porridge warm, garnished with sliced almonds if desired.

Nutrition (per serving):

- Calories: 220

- Protein: 4g

- Carbohydrates: 43g

- Fat: 4g

- Fiber: 1g

Preparation Time: 10 minutes

Cooking Time: 10 minutes

Servings: 2 (6 small pancakes)

Ingredients:

- 1 ripe banana, mashed

- 2 large eggs

- 1/2 teaspoon vanilla extract

- 1/2 cup whole wheat flour

- 1/2 teaspoon baking powder

- Pinch of salt

- Cooking spray or a small amount of oil for greasing the pan

Directions:

1. In a bowl, whisk together the mashed banana, eggs, and vanilla extract until well combined.

2. In a separate bowl, mix the whole wheat flour, baking powder, and salt.

3. Add the dry ingredients to the wet ingredients and stir until just combined. Do not overmix.

4. Heat a non-stick skillet or griddle over medium heat. Lightly coat with cooking spray or a small amount of oil.

5. Pour 1/4 cup of the pancake batter onto the skillet for each pancake.

6. Cook for 2-3 minutes, until bubbles start to form on the surface. Flip the pancakes and cook for an additional 1-2 minutes until golden brown.

7. Repeat with the remaining batter.

8. Serve the banana pancakes warm with desired toppings such as fresh berries or a drizzle of honey.

Nutrition (per serving, 3 small pancakes):

- Calories: 200

- Protein: 8g

- Carbohydrates: 33g

- Fat: 5g

- Fiber: 4g

Greek Yogurt with Honey and Strawberries:

Preparation Time: 5 minutes

Servings: 1

Ingredients:

- 1/2 cup Greek yogurt

- 1 tablespoon honey or a low-sugar sweetener

- 1/2 cup fresh strawberries, sliced

Directions:

1. In a bowl, spoon the Greek yogurt.

2. Drizzle honey over the yogurt.

3. Top with sliced strawberries.

4. Gently mix the ingredients together.

5. Enjoy the Greek yogurt with honey and strawberries as a nutritious and refreshing snack or breakfast option.

Nutrition (per serving):

- Calories: 150

- Protein: 12g

- Carbohydrates: 23g

- Fat: 2g

- Fiber: 2g

Avocado Toast on Whole Grain Bread:

Preparation Time: 5 minutes

Servings: 1

Ingredients:

- 1 slice of whole grain bread, toasted

- 1/2 ripe avocado

- Pinch of salt

- Pinch of black pepper

- Optional toppings: sliced tomatoes, sprouts, or a squeeze of lemon juice

Directions:

1. Toast the slice of whole grain bread until golden brown.

2. Cut the ripe avocado in half, remove the pit, and scoop the flesh into a bowl.

3. Mash the avocado with a fork until smooth.

4. Spread the mashed avocado onto the toasted bread.

5. Sprinkle with a pinch of salt and black pepper.

6. Add optional toppings, such as sliced tomatoes, sprouts, or a squeeze of lemon juice, if desired.

7. Serve the avocado toast as a healthy and satisfying breakfast or snack.

Nutrition (per serving):

- Calories: 200

- Protein: 5g

- Carbohydrates: 20g

- Fat: 12g

- Fiber: 7g

Preparation Time: 5 minutes

Cooking Time: 20 minutes

Servings: 2

Ingredients:

- 1/2 cup quinoa, rinsed

- 1 cup water

- 1/2 cup fresh or frozen blueberries

- 1 tablespoon honey or a low-sugar sweetener

- 1/4 teaspoon vanilla extract

- Optional toppings: sliced almonds, shredded coconut, or a sprinkle of cinnamon

Directions:

1. In a saucepan, combine the rinsed quinoa and water. Bring to a boil over medium heat.

2. Reduce the heat to low, cover the saucepan, and simmer for about 15-20 minutes, or until the quinoa is cooked and the water is absorbed.

3. Remove from heat and let it sit covered for 5 minutes.

4. Fluff the quinoa with a fork.

5. Stir in the blueberries, honey, and vanilla extract.

6. Serve the blueberry breakfast quinoa warm, and add optional toppings such as sliced almonds, shredded coconut, or a sprinkle of cinnamon for extra flavor and texture.

Nutrition (per serving):

- Calories: 200

- Protein: 6g

- Carbohydrates: 39g

- Fat: 3g

- Fiber: 4g

Spiced Pear Compote:

Preparation Time: 10 minutes

Cooking Time: 15 minutes

Servings: 2

Ingredients:

- 2 ripe pears, peeled, cored, and diced

- 1 tablespoon honey or a low-sugar sweetener

- 1/2 teaspoon ground cinnamon

- 1/4 teaspoon ground ginger

- Pinch of nutmeg

- 1/4 cup water

- 1 tablespoon lemon juice

Directions:

1. In a saucepan, combine the diced pears, honey, ground cinnamon, ground ginger, nutmeg, water, and lemon juice.

2. Cook over medium heat, stirring occasionally, for about 10-15 minutes, or until the pears are tender and the mixture has thickened.

3. Remove from heat and let it cool slightly.

4. Serve the spiced pear compote warm as a topping for oatmeal, yogurt, pancakes, or toast.

Nutrition (per serving):

- Calories: 80

- Protein: 1g

- Carbohydrates: 21g

- Fat: 0g

- Fiber: 4g

Tofu Scramble with Vegetables:

Preparation Time: 10 minutes

Cooking Time: 15 minutes

Servings: 2

Ingredients:

- 8 ounces firm tofu, drained and crumbled

- 1 tablespoon olive oil

- 1/2 small onion, diced

- 1/2 bell pepper, diced

- 1/2 cup sliced mushrooms

- 1/2 cup spinach leaves

- 1/2 teaspoon ground turmeric

- 1/2 teaspoon ground cumin

- Salt and pepper to taste

- Optional toppings: diced tomatoes, avocado slices, or chopped fresh herbs

Directions:

1. Heat olive oil in a skillet over medium heat.

2. Add the diced onion, bell pepper, and mushrooms to the skillet. Sauté for 5 minutes until the vegetables are tender.

3. Add the crumbled tofu, ground turmeric, ground cumin, salt, and pepper to the skillet. Stir well to combine.

4. Cook for another 5-7 minutes, stirring occasionally, until the tofu is heated through and lightly browned.

5. Add the spinach leaves and cook for an additional 2 minutes until wilted.

6. Remove from heat and serve the tofu scramble hot.

7. Top with optional toppings such as diced tomatoes, avocado slices, or chopped fresh herbs for added freshness and flavor.

Nutrition (per serving):

- Calories: 150

- Protein: 12g

- Carbohydrates: 8g

- Fat: 9g

- Fiber: 3g

Preparation Time: 10 minutes

Cooking Time: 20 minutes

Servings: 2

Ingredients:

- 1 large sweet potato, peeled and grated

- 1/2 small onion, finely diced

- 1 tablespoon olive oil

- 1/2 teaspoon paprika

- 1/4 teaspoon garlic powder

- Salt and pepper to taste

Directions:

1. Place the grated sweet potato in a clean kitchen towel and squeeze out any excess moisture.

2. In a large bowl, combine the grated sweet potato, diced onion, paprika, garlic powder, salt, and pepper. Mix well.

3. Heat olive oil in a skillet over medium heat.

4. Add the sweet potato mixture to the skillet, pressing it down gently to form a layer.

5. Cook for about 10-12 minutesuntil the bottom is golden brown.

6. Carefully flip the hash browns using a spatula and cook for another 8-10 minutes until the other side is golden brown and crispy.

7. Remove from heat and serve the sweet potato hash browns hot as a delicious and nutritious breakfast side dish.

Nutrition (per serving):

- Calories: 150

- Protein: 2g

- Carbohydrates: 20g

- Fat: 7g

- Fiber: 4g

Cranberry Almond Breakfast Bars:

Preparation Time: 15 minutes

Cooking Time: 25 minutes

Servings: 9 bars

Ingredients:

- 1 1/2 cups old-fashioned oats

- 1/2 cup almond flour

- 1/4 cup dried cranberries

- 1/4 cup sliced almonds

- 1/4 cup honey or a low-sugar sweetener

- 2 tablespoons almond butter

- 1 tablespoon melted coconut oil

- 1/2 teaspoon vanilla extract

- 1/4 teaspoon salt

Directions:

1. Preheat the oven to 350°F (175°C). Grease or line an 8x8-inch baking dish with parchment paper.

2. In a large bowl, mix together the oats, almond flour, dried cranberries, and sliced almonds.

3. In a separate microwave-safe bowl, combine the honey, almond butter, melted coconut oil, vanilla extract, and salt. Microwave for 20-30 seconds, or until the mixture is warm and easily stirrable.

4. Pour the wet ingredients over the dry ingredients and stir until well combined.

5. Transfer the mixture to the prepared baking dish and press it down firmly.

6. Bake for 20-25 minutes, or until the edges are golden brown.

7. Remove from the oven and let it cool completely before cutting into bars.

8. Store the cranberry almond breakfast bars in an airtight container for up to one week.

Nutrition (per bar):

- Calories: 170

- Protein: 4g

- Carbohydrates: 22g

- Fat: 8g

- Fiber: 3g

Pumpkin Spice Overnight Oats:

Preparation Time: 5 minutes

Chilling Time: Overnight

Servings: 2

Ingredients:

- 1 cup rolled oats

- 1 cup unsweetened almond milk (or any milk of your choice)

- 1/2 cup pumpkin puree

- 1 tablespoon maple syrup or a low-sugar sweetener

- 1/2 teaspoon pumpkin pie spice

- Optional toppings: chopped nuts, raisins, or a sprinkle of cinnamon

Directions:

1. In a bowl or jar, combine the rolled oats, almond milk, pumpkin puree, maple syrup, and pumpkin pie spice. Stir well to combine.

2. Cover the bowl or jar and refrigerate overnight or for at least 4 hours.

3. In the morning, give the overnight oats a good stir.

4. Serve the pumpkin spice overnight oats cold or warmed up in the microwave.

5. Top with optional toppings such as chopped nuts, raisins, or a sprinkle of cinnamon for added texture and flavor.

Nutrition (per serving):

- Calories: 220

- Protein: 7g

- Carbohydrates: 38g

- Fat: 5g

- Fiber: 7g

Lemon Poppy Seed Scones:

Preparation Time: 15 minutes

Cooking Time: 15 minutes

Servings: 8 scones

Ingredients:

- 2 cups all-purpose flour

- 1/4 cup granulated sugar

- 2 teaspoons baking powder

- 1/2 teaspoon baking soda

- 1/4 teaspoon salt

- Zest of 1 lemon

- 1 tablespoon poppy seeds

- 1/2 cup unsalted butter, cold and cubed

- 1/2 cup buttermilk (or 1/2 cup milk mixed with 1/2 tablespoon lemon juice)

- 1 tablespoon lemon juice

- 1 teaspoon vanilla extract

- Optional glaze: powdered sugar mixed with lemon juice

Directions:

1. Preheat the oven to 400°F (200°C). Line a baking sheet with parchment paper.

2. In a large bowl, whisk together the flour, sugar, baking powder, baking soda, salt, lemon zest, and poppy seeds.

3. Add the cold cubed butter to the dry ingredients. Using a pastry cutter or your fingers, cut the butter into the flour mixture until it resembles coarse crumbs.

4. In a separate bowl, whisk together the buttermilk, lemon juice, and vanilla extract.

5. Pour the wet ingredients into the dry ingredients. Stir until just combined and a dough forms. Be careful not to overmix.

6. Transfer the dough onto a lightly floured surface. Gently pat the dough into a circle about 1-inch thick.

7. Cut the dough into 8 wedges and place them on the prepared baking sheet.

8. Bake for 12-15 minutes, or until the scones are golden brown.

9. Remove from the oven and let them cool on a wire rack.

10. Optional: Drizzle the cooled scones with a glaze made from powdered sugar mixed with lemon juice.

11. Serve the lemon poppy seed scones with a cup oftea or coffee.

Nutrition (per scone):

- Calories: 240

- Protein: 4g

- Carbohydrates: 30g

- Fat: 11g

- Fiber: 1g

Coconut Chia Seed Pudding:

Preparation Time: 5 minutes

Chilling Time: 2 hours or overnight

Servings: 2

Ingredients:

- 1/4 cup chia seeds

- 1 cup coconut milk (canned or carton)

- 1 tablespoon maple syrup or a low-sugar sweetener

- 1/2 teaspoon vanilla extract

- Optional toppings: fresh berries, shredded coconut, or chopped nuts

Directions:

1. In a bowl or jar, combine the chia seeds, coconut milk, maple syrup, and vanilla extract. Stir well to combine.

2. Cover the bowl or jar and refrigerate for at least 2 hours or overnight. Stir the mixture after the first hour to prevent clumping.

3. Once the chia seed pudding has thickened to a pudding-like consistency, give it a good stir.

4. Serve the coconut chia seed pudding cold.

5. Top with optional toppings such as fresh berries, shredded coconut, or chopped nuts for added texture and flavor.

Nutrition (per serving):

- Calories: 220

- Protein: 5g

- Carbohydrates: 16g

- Fat: 16g

- Fiber: 10g

<table><tr><td>

Herbal Tea with Lemon:

</td></tr></table>

Preparation Time: 5 minutes

Steeping Time: 5 minutes

Servings: 1

Ingredients:

- 1 herbal tea bag (such as chamomile, peppermint, or ginger)

- 1 cup boiling water

- Fresh lemon slices

- Honey or a low-sugar sweetener (optional)

Directions:

1. Place the herbal tea bag in a mug.

2. Pour the boiling water over the tea bag and let it steep for 5 minutes.

3. Remove the tea bag and add fresh lemon slices.

4. Sweeten with honey or a low-sugar sweetener, if desired.

5. Stir well and enjoy the herbal tea with lemon while it's still warm.

Note: Feel free to experiment with different herbal tea flavors and adjust the steeping time according to package instructions for optimal taste.

Poached Eggs on English Muffins:

Preparation Time: 10 minutes

Cooking Time: 5 minutes

Servings: 2

Ingredients:

- 4 large eggs

- 2 English muffins, split and toasted

- Butter or olive oil, for spreading

- Salt and pepper, to taste

- Optional toppings: avocado slices, smoked salmon, or fresh herbs

Directions:

1. Fill a large saucepan with water, about 2-3 inches deep. Bring the water to a gentle simmer over medium heat.

2. Crack each egg into a small bowl or ramekin, taking care not to break the yolks.

3. Create a gentle whirlpool in the simmering water using a spoon or spatula.

4. Carefully slide one egg into the center of the whirlpool. Repeat with the remaining eggs, cooking them one at a time.

5. Poach the eggs for about 3-4 minutes for a runny yolk or 5-6 minutes for a firmer yolk.

6. While the eggs are poaching, spread butter or olive oil on the toasted English muffins.

7. Once the eggs are done, carefully remove them from the water using a slotted spoon and drain off any excess water.

8. Place one poached egg on each English muffin half.

9. Sprinkle with salt and pepper to taste.

10. Add optional toppings such as avocado slices, smoked salmon, or fresh herbs.

11. Serve the poached eggs on English muffins immediately.

Cinnamon Raisin Bread:

Preparation Time: 2 hours 30 minutes

Cooking Time: 40 minutes

Servings: 1 loaf

Ingredients:

- 2 cups all-purpose flour

- 1/4 cup granulated sugar

- 2 teaspoons active dry yeast

- 1/2 teaspoon salt

- 1/2 teaspoon ground cinnamon

- 3/4 cup warm milk

- 2 tablespoons unsalted butter, melted

- 1/2 cup raisins

For the filling:

- 2 tablespoons unsalted butter, softened

- 1/4 cup granulated sugar

- 1 teaspoon ground cinnamon

For the glaze:

- 1/2 cup powdered sugar

- 1-2 tablespoons milk

- 1/2 teaspoon vanilla extract

Directions:

1. In a large bowl, combine the flour, sugar, yeast, salt, and ground cinnamon.

2. In a separate bowl, mix together the warm milk and melted butter.

3. Pour the milk mixture into the dry ingredients. Stir until a dough forms.

4. Transfer the dough to a floured surface and knead for about 5 minutes, or until smooth and elastic.

5. Place the dough in a greased bowl, cover with a clean kitchen towel, and let it rise in a warm place for 1-1.5 hours, or until doubled in size.

6. Meanwhile, prepare the filling by combining the softened butter, granulated sugar, and ground cinnamon in a small bowl. Set aside.

7. Once the dough has risen, punch it down to release the air. Roll it out into a rectangle shape on a floured surface.

8. Spread the filling evenly over the dough, leaving a small border around the edges. Sprinkle the raisins on top of the filling.

9. Starting from one of the longer sides, tightly roll up the dough into a log shape.

10. Place the rolled dough into a greased loaf pan. Cover with the kitchen towel and let it rise for another 30-45 minutes.

11. Preheat the oven to 350°F (175°C).

12. Bake the cinnamon raisin bread for 35-40 minutes, or until golden brown and cooked through.

13. Remove from the oven and let it cool in the pan for a few minutes. Then transfer the bread to a wire rack to cool completely.

14. In a small bowl, whisk together the powdered sugar, milk, and vanilla extract to make the glaze.

15. Drizzle the glaze over the cooledcinnamon raisin bread.

16. Slice the bread and serve it as desired. It can be enjoyed plain or toasted with butter.

Vanilla Rice Pudding:

Preparation Time: 5 minutes

Cooking Time: 30 minutes

Chilling Time: 2 hours (optional)

Servings: 4-6

Ingredients:

- 1 cup white rice

- 4 cups milk (whole or 2%)

- 1/2 cup granulated sugar

- 1 teaspoon vanilla extract

- Ground cinnamon, for garnish (optional)

Directions:

1. Rinse the rice under cold water to remove excess starch.

2. In a large saucepan, combine the rinsed rice, milk, and sugar.

3. Place the saucepan over medium heat and bring the mixture to a gentle boil, stirring occasionally.

4. Reduce the heat to low and let the rice simmer, stirring occasionally, for about 25-30 minutes or until the rice is tender and the mixture has thickened.

5. Remove the saucepan from the heat and stir in the vanilla extract.

6. If preferred, you can chill the rice pudding in the refrigerator for a couple of hours to serve it cold. Otherwise, you can serve it warm immediately.

7. Before serving, sprinkle ground cinnamon on top for added flavor and garnish, if desired.

8. Spoon the vanilla rice pudding into serving bowls or glasses.

9. Enjoy the rice pudding warm or chilled, depending on your preference.

Note: You can customize the rice pudding by adding raisins, chopped nuts, or a sprinkle of nutmeg. Feel free to adjust the sweetness to your liking by adding more or less sugar.

Chapter 3:

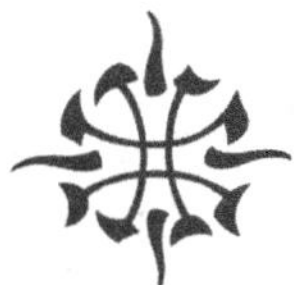

LIGHT LUNCHES

Chicken Salad with Apples and Walnuts:

Preparation Time: 15 minutes

Cooking Time: 20 minutes

Servings: 4

Ingredients:

- 2 boneless, skinless chicken breasts

- 1 apple, cored and diced

- 1/2 cup walnuts, chopped

- 1/4 cup red onion, finely chopped

- 1/4 cup plain Greek yogurt

- 1 tablespoon lemon juice

- 1 tablespoon Dijon mustard

- Salt and pepper to taste

- Lettuce leaves, for serving

Directions:

1. Preheat your grill or stovetop grill pan over medium heat.

2. Season the chicken breasts with salt and pepper.

3. Grill the chicken for about 8-10 minutes on each side, or until cooked through. Let it rest for a few minutes before slicing it into thin strips.

4. In a large bowl, combine the diced apple, chopped walnuts, red onion, Greek yogurt, lemon juice, and Dijon mustard. Mix well.

5. Add the sliced chicken to the bowl and toss gently to coat the chicken with the dressing.

6. Taste and adjust the seasoning with salt and pepper if needed.

7. Serve the chicken salad on a bed of lettuce leaves or as a filling for sandwiches or wraps.

Nutrition:

- This chicken salad is a nutritious option, providing lean protein from the chicken, healthy fats from walnuts, and fiber from apples.

- The Greek yogurt adds creaminess without excessive fat, and the lemon juice and Dijon mustard provide a tangy flavor.

- Remember to keep portion sizes in mind, as the nutritional content may vary based on the specific brands and quantities of ingredients used.

Lentil Soup with Carrots and Celery:

Preparation Time: 10 minutes

Cooking Time: 45 minutes

Servings: 6

Ingredients:

- 1 cup dried lentils, rinsed and drained

- 1 onion, chopped

- 2 carrots, diced

- 2 celery stalks, diced

- 2 cloves garlic, minced

- 4 cups low-sodium vegetable broth

- 1 bay leaf

- 1 teaspoon dried thyme

- Salt and pepper to taste

- Fresh parsley for garnish (optional)

Directions:

1. In a large pot, sauté the chopped onion, carrots, celery, and minced garlic over medium heat until they soften, about 5 minutes.

2. Add the rinsed lentils, vegetable broth, bay leaf, dried thyme, salt, and pepper to the pot. Stir well.

3. Bring the soup to a boil, then reduce the heat to low and let it simmer for about 40 minutes, or until the lentils are tender.

4. Remove the bay leaf from the pot.

5. If desired, use an immersion blender to blend a portion of the soup until smooth, or leave it chunky for a heartier texture.

6. Adjust the seasoning with salt and pepper to taste.

7. Serve the lentil soup hot, garnished with fresh parsley if desired.

Nutrition:

- Lentils are an excellent source of plant-based protein and dietary fiber, making this soup both satisfying and nourishing.

- Carrots and celery add vitamins and minerals, while the low-sodium vegetable broth keeps the sodium content in check.

- The soup is low in fat and can be enjoyed as a main course or as a side dish.

Turkey and Avocado Wrap:

Preparation Time: 10 minutes

Servings: 2

Ingredients:

- 4 large lettuce leaves

- 8 ounces deli turkey breast slices

- 1 avocado, sliced

- 1/2 cup cherry tomatoes, halved

- 2 tablespoons mayonnaise or Greek yogurt

- Salt and pepper to taste

Directions:

1. Lay the lettuce leaves flat on a clean surface.

2. Spread a tablespoon of mayonnaise or Greek yogurt over each lettuce leaf.

3. Divide the turkey breast slices evenly among the lettuce leaves.

4. Top the turkey with avocado slices and cherry tomato halves.

5. Season with salt and pepper to taste.

6. Roll up each lettuce leaf tightly to form a wrap.

7. Slice the wraps in half diagonally and secure with toothpicks if needed.

8. Serve the turkey and avocado wraps as a light and refreshing meal or pack them for a convenient on-the-go lunch.

Nutrition:

- This turkey and avocado wrap offers a balanced combination of lean protein from the turkey, healthy fats from avocado, and fresh vegetables.

- Lettuce acts as a low-calorie alternative to traditional bread or tortilla wraps.

- Adjust the amount of mayonnaise or Greek yogurt according to personal preference, keeping in mind that excessive amounts can increase calorie and fat content.

Quinoa Salad with Cucumber and Tomato:

Preparation Time: 15 minutes

Cooking Time: 15 minutes

Servings:4

Ingredients:

- 1 cup quinoa, rinsed

- 2 cups water

- 1 cucumber, diced

- 1 cup cherry tomatoes, halved

- 1/4 cup red onion, finely chopped

- 1/4 cup fresh parsley, chopped

- 2 tablespoons extra-virgin olive oil

- 2 tablespoons lemon juice

- Salt and pepper to taste

Directions:

1. In a medium saucepan, bring the water to a boil. Add the rinsed quinoa and reduce the heat to low. Cover and simmer for about 15 minutes, or until the quinoa is cooked and the water is absorbed. Remove from heat and let it cool.

2. In a large bowl, combine the cooked quinoa, diced cucumber, cherry tomatoes, red onion, and fresh parsley.

3. In a separate small bowl, whisk together the extra-virgin olive oil and lemon juice to make the dressing.

4. Pour the dressing over the quinoa salad and toss gently to coat all the ingredients.

5. Season with salt and pepper to taste.

6. Let the salad sit for a few minutes to allow the flavors to meld together.

7. Serve the quinoa salad as a refreshing side dish or a light meal on its own.

Nutrition:

- Quinoa is a nutritious grain that provides a good source of plant-based protein, dietary fiber, and essential minerals.

- Cucumber and tomatoes add freshness and hydration to the salad, while red onion and parsley contribute to its flavor and nutritional profile.

- The dressing made with extra-virgin olive oil and lemon juice adds a tangy taste and healthy fats.

- Adjust the seasoning and dressing quantities according to personal preference, keeping in mind the overall nutritional goals.

Tuna Salad with Greek Yogurt:

Preparation Time: 10 minutes

Servings: 2

Ingredients:

- 1 can (5 ounces) tuna, drained

- 1/4 cup diced celery

- 1/4 cup diced red onion

- 1/4 cup diced pickles

- 2 tablespoons plain Greek yogurt

- 1 tablespoon lemon juice

- 1 teaspoon Dijon mustard

- Salt and pepper to taste

- Lettuce leaves, for serving

Directions:

1. In a medium bowl, flake the drained tuna using a fork.

2. Add the diced celery, red onion, and pickles to the bowl and mix well.

3. In a small bowl, whisk together the Greek yogurt, lemon juice, Dijon mustard, salt, and pepper.

4. Pour the dressing over the tuna mixture and toss gently until well combined.

5. Taste and adjust the seasoning as needed.

6. Serve the tuna salad on a bed of lettuce leaves or use it as a filling for sandwiches or wraps.

Nutrition:

- This tuna salad offers a protein-rich meal option, with Greek yogurt providing a creamy texture without excess fat.

- Celery, red onion, and pickles add crunch and flavor while keeping the sodium content under control.

- Adjust the quantities of ingredients and dressing according to personal preferences and dietary restrictions.

Preparation Time: 10 minutes

Cooking Time: 25 minutes

Servings: 4

Ingredients:

- 1 tablespoon olive oil

- 1 onion, chopped

- 3 cloves garlic, minced

- 1 teaspoon ground cumin

- 1/2 teaspoon ground coriander

- 1/4 teaspoon turmeric

- 1 can (15 ounces) chickpeas, rinsed and drained

- 1 can (14 ounces) diced tomatoes

- 2 cups vegetable broth

- 4 cups fresh spinach leaves

- Salt and pepper to taste

Directions:

1. Heat the olive oil in a large pot over medium heat.

2. Add the chopped onion and minced garlic to the pot and sauté until the onion becomes translucent, about 5 minutes.

3. Stir in the ground cumin, ground coriander, and turmeric, and cook for an additional minute to toast the spices.

4. Add the chickpeas, diced tomatoes (with their juices), and vegetable broth to the pot. Stir well to combine.

5. Bring the mixture to a boil, then reduce the heat to low and let it simmer for about 15 minutes to allow the flavors to meld together.

6. Add the fresh spinach leaves to the pot and stir until they wilt and become tender, about 2-3 minutes.

7. Season the stew with salt and pepper to taste.

8. Serve the chickpea and spinach stew hot as a satisfying and nutritious meal.

Nutrition:

- This stew combines protein-rich chickpeas with nutrient-dense spinach, providing a well-rounded meal option.

- The spices add flavor and depth to the dish, while the vegetable broth keeps the sodium content controlled.

- Adjust the spices and seasoning according to personal taste preferences.

Grilled Chicken and Mango Salad:

Preparation Time: 15 minutes

Cooking Time: 15 minutes

Servings: 2

Ingredients:

- 2 boneless, skinless chicken breasts

- 1 mango, peeled and diced

- 1/2 red bell pepper, diced

- 1/4 cup red onion, finely chopped

- 2 tablespoons chopped fresh cilantro

- 1 tablespoon lime juice

- 1 tablespoon olive oil

- Salt and pepper to taste

- Mixed salad greens, for serving

Directions:

1. Preheat your grill or stovetop grill pan over medium heat.

2. Season the chicken breasts with salt and pepper.

3. Grill the chicken for about 6-8 minutes on each side, or until cooked through. Let it rest for a few minutes before slicing it into thin strips.

4. In a large bowl, combine the diced mango, red bell pepper, red onion, chopped cilantro, lime juice, olive oil, salt, and pepper. Toss well to combine.

5. Add the sliced grilled chicken to the bowl and gently mix it with the mango salad.

6. Taste and adjust the seasoning as needed.

7. Serve the grilled chicken and mango salad on a bed of mixed salad greens for a refreshing and satisfying meal.

Nutrition:

- This salad offers a balance of lean protein from the grilled chicken, natural sweetness from mango, and a variety of vibrant vegetables.

- The lime juice and cilantro add a zesty and refreshing flavor, while the olive oil provides a healthy source of fat.

- Adjust the quantities of ingredients and dressing according to personal preferences and dietary needs.

Cucumber and Dill Sandwiches:

Preparation Time: 10 minutes

Servings: 2

Ingredients:

- 4 slices of bread (whole wheat or your choice)

- 1 large cucumber, thinly sliced

- 4 tablespoons cream cheese

- 2 tablespoons fresh dill, chopped

- Salt and pepper to taste

Directions:

1. Spread cream cheese evenly on all four slices of bread.

2. Arrange the thinly sliced cucumber on two of the bread slices.

3. Sprinkle chopped dill over the cucumber slices.

4. Season with salt and pepper to taste.

5. Place the remaining two slices of bread on top to make sandwiches.

6. Press the sandwiches gently to hold them together.

7. Cut the sandwiches into desired shapes, such as triangles or rectangles, if desired.

8. Serve the cucumber and dill sandwiches as a light and refreshing snack or lunch option.

Nutrition:

- These cucumber and dill sandwiches are a low-calorie option with fresh and crisp cucumber providing hydration and fiber.

- Cream cheese adds a creamy and tangy element, while dill offers a refreshing flavor.

- Choose whole wheat bread for added fiber and nutrients.

- Adjust the quantities and types of ingredients according to personal preferences and dietary needs.

Tomato Basil Soup

Preparation Time: 10 minutes

Cooking Time: 30 minutes

Servings: 4

Ingredients:

- 4 large tomatoes, chopped

- 1 small onion, chopped

- 2 cloves garlic, minced

- 1 cup low-sodium vegetable broth

- 1/2 cup fresh basil leaves, chopped

- 1 tablespoon olive oil

- 1/2 teaspoon salt (optional)

- 1/4 teaspoon black pepper

- 1/4 cup plain Greek yogurt (optional for creaminess)

Directions:

1. Heat the olive oil in a large pot over medium heat. Add the onion and garlic, sautéing until softened, about 5 minutes.

2. Add the chopped tomatoes and cook for another 5 minutes, stirring occasionally.

3. Pour in the vegetable broth and bring the mixture to a boil. Reduce the heat and let it simmer for 20 minutes.

4. Add the basil leaves and blend the soup using an immersion blender until smooth. If you prefer a creamier soup, stir in the Greek yogurt.

5. Season with salt and pepper to taste. Serve hot.

Nutrition (per serving):

- Calories: 90

- Protein: 2g

- Carbohydrates: 12g

- Fat: 4g

- Sodium: 150mg

- Potassium: 400mg

Egg Salad with Low-Fat Mayo

Preparation Time: 15 minutes

Cooking Time: 10 minutes

Servings: 4

Ingredients:

- 6 large eggs

- 1/4 cup low-fat mayonnaise

- 1 teaspoon Dijon mustard

- 1 small celery stalk, finely chopped

- 1 tablespoon fresh chives, chopped

- 1/4 teaspoon salt (optional)

- 1/4 teaspoon black pepper

Directions:

1. Place the eggs in a pot and cover with water. Bring to a boil, then reduce the heat and simmer for 10 minutes.

2. Drain the hot water and place the eggs in a bowl of ice water to cool. Peel the eggs once they are cool.

3. Chop the eggs and place them in a mixing bowl. Add the low-fat mayonnaise, Dijon mustard, celery, and chives.

4. Mix everything until well combined. Season with salt and pepper to taste.

5. Serve immediately or refrigerate until ready to use.

Nutrition (per serving):

- Calories: 150

- Protein: 9g

- Carbohydrates: 2g

- Fat: 11g

- Sodium: 200mg

- Potassium: 120mg

Barley and Vegetable Soup

Preparation Time: 15 minutes

Cooking Time: 45 minutes

Servings: 6

Ingredients:

- 1 cup barley

- 1 medium carrot, chopped

- 1 celery stalk, chopped

- 1 small onion, chopped

- 2 cloves garlic, minced

- 1 cup diced tomatoes (no salt added)

- 4 cups low-sodium vegetable broth

- 1 tablespoon olive oil

- 1 teaspoon dried thyme

- 1/2 teaspoon dried basil

- 1/4 teaspoon black pepper

Directions:

1. Heat the olive oil in a large pot over medium heat. Add the onion, carrot, celery, and garlic, sautéing until softened, about 5 minutes.

2. Add the barley and cook for another 2 minutes, stirring constantly.

3. Pour in the vegetable broth and diced tomatoes. Bring the mixture to a boil.

4. Reduce the heat and let it simmer for 45 minutes, or until the barley is tender.

5. Stir in the thyme, basil, and black pepper. Serve hot.

Nutrition (per serving):

- Calories: 180

- Protein: 4g

- Carbohydrates: 35g

- Fat: 3g

- Sodium: 150mg

- Potassium: 350mg

Roasted Red Pepper Hummus Wrap

Preparation Time: 15 minutes

Cooking Time: 10 minutes

Servings: 4

Ingredients:

- 1 cup roasted red peppers, chopped

- 1 can (15 oz) chickpeas, drained and rinsed

- 1/4 cup tahini

- 2 tablespoons lemon juice

- 1 garlic clove, minced

- 1/2 teaspoon cumin

- 4 whole wheat tortillas

- 1 cup fresh spinach leaves

- 1/2 cup shredded carrots

- 1/4 teaspoon salt (optional)

- 1/4 teaspoon black pepper

Directions:

1. In a food processor, combine the chickpeas, roasted red peppers, tahini, lemon juice, garlic, and cumin. Blend until smooth. Season with salt and pepper to taste.

2. Spread a generous amount of hummus onto each whole wheat tortilla.

3. Layer the spinach leaves and shredded carrots on top of the hummus.

4. Roll up the tortillas, slice in half, and serve.

Nutrition (per serving):

- Calories: 250

- Protein: 8g

- Carbohydrates: 36g

- Fat: 8g

- Sodium: 200mg

- Potassium: 300mg

Stuffed Bell Peppers with Quinoa

Preparation Time: 20 minutes

Cooking Time: 40 minutes

Servings: 4

Ingredients:

- 4 large bell peppers (any color), tops cut off and seeds removed

- 1 cup quinoa

- 2 cups low-sodium vegetable broth

- 1 small onion, chopped

- 1 medium zucchini, chopped

- 1 cup diced tomatoes (no salt added)

- 1/2 cup black beans, drained and rinsed

- 1 tablespoon olive oil

- 1 teaspoon cumin

- 1/2 teaspoon paprika

- 1/4 teaspoon black pepper

- 1/4 cup chopped fresh parsley

Directions:

1. Preheat the oven to 375°F (190°C). Cook the quinoa in vegetable broth according to package instructions, then set aside.

2. In a large skillet, heat the olive oil over medium heat. Add the onion and zucchini, sautéing until softened, about 5 minutes.

3. Stir in the diced tomatoes, black beans, cumin, paprika, and black pepper. Cook for another 5 minutes, then mix in the cooked quinoa.

4. Spoon the quinoa mixture into the hollowed bell peppers, filling them completely.

5. Place the stuffed peppers in a baking dish and cover with foil. Bake for 30 minutes, then remove the foil and bake for an additional 10 minutes.

6. Garnish with chopped fresh parsley and serve.

Nutrition (per serving):

- Calories: 220

- Protein: 8g

- Carbohydrates: 38g

- Fat: 6g

- Sodium: 120mg

- Potassium: 450mg

Cold Zucchini Noodles with Pesto

Preparation Time: 15 minutes

Cooking Time: None

Servings: 4

Ingredients:

- 4 medium zucchinis, spiralized into noodles

- 1 cup fresh basil leaves

- 1/4 cup pine nuts

- 1/4 cup grated Parmesan cheese

- 1/4 cup olive oil

- 1 garlic clove

- 1 tablespoon lemon juice

- 1/4 teaspoon salt (optional)

- 1/4 teaspoon black pepper

Directions:

1. In a food processor, combine the basil leaves, pine nuts, Parmesan cheese, garlic, lemon juice, salt, and black pepper. Blend until smooth.

2. With the food processor running, gradually add the olive oil until the pesto reaches a smooth consistency.

3. Toss the zucchini noodles with the pesto until evenly coated.

4. Serve immediately, or chill in the refrigerator for a more refreshing dish.

Nutrition (per serving):

- Calories: 200

- Protein: 5g

- Carbohydrates: 8g

- Fat: 18g

- Sodium: 150mg

- Potassium: 400mg

Beet and Orange Salad

Preparation Time: 15 minutes

Cooking Time: None

Servings: 4

Ingredients:

- 4 medium beets, cooked and sliced

- 2 large oranges, peeled and segmented

- 1/4 cup red onion, thinly sliced

- 1/4 cup fresh mint leaves, chopped

- 2 tablespoons olive oil

- 1 tablespoon balsamic vinegar

- 1/4 teaspoon salt (optional)

- 1/4 teaspoon black pepper

Directions:

1. In a large bowl, combine the sliced beets, orange segments, and red onion.

2. In a small bowl, whisk together the olive oil, balsamic vinegar, salt, and black pepper.

3. Drizzle the dressing over the salad and toss gently to combine.

4. Garnish with chopped mint leaves and serve immediately.

Nutrition (per serving):

- Calories: 150

- Protein: 2g

- Carbohydrates: 18g

- Fat: 7g

- Sodium: 100mg

- Potassium: 450mg

Cauliflower Rice Stir-Fry

Preparation Time: 15 minutes

Cooking Time: 15 minutes

Servings: 4

Ingredients:

- 1 large head of cauliflower, grated into rice-sized pieces

- 1 cup frozen peas and carrots, thawed

- 1 small bell pepper, chopped

- 1 small onion, chopped

- 2 cloves garlic, minced

- 2 tablespoons low-sodium soy sauce

- 1 tablespoon olive oil

- 1/2 teaspoon ginger powder

- 1/4 teaspoon black pepper

- 2 green onions, chopped

Directions:

1. Heat the olive oil in a large skillet over medium heat. Add the onion and garlic, sautéing until fragrant, about 3 minutes.

2. Add the bell pepper, peas, and carrots, cooking for another 5 minutes until the vegetables are tender.

3. Stir in the grated cauliflower, soy sauce, ginger powder, and black pepper. Cook for an additional 5 minutes, stirring occasionally, until the cauliflower is tender but not mushy.

4. Garnish with chopped green onions and serve hot.

Nutrition (per serving):

- Calories: 120

- Protein: 4g

- Carbohydrates: 15g

- Fat: 5g

- Sodium: 220mg

- Potassium: 350mg

Broccoli Cheddar Soup

Preparation Time: 15 minutes

Cooking Time: 30 minutes

Servings: 4

Ingredients:

- 1 large head of broccoli, chopped into florets

- 1 small onion, chopped

- 2 cloves garlic, minced

- 2 cups low-sodium vegetable broth

- 1 cup low-fat milk

- 1 cup shredded low-fat cheddar cheese

- 1 tablespoon olive oil

- 2 tablespoons all-purpose flour

- 1/4 teaspoon black pepper

- 1/4 teaspoon paprika

Directions:

1. Heat the olive oil in a large pot over medium heat. Add the onion and garlic, sautéing until softened, about 5 minutes.

2. Stir in the flour and cook for another minute, stirring constantly.

3. Slowly whisk in the vegetable broth and milk, bringing the mixture to a simmer.

4. Add the chopped broccoli and cook for 15 minutes, until tender.

5. Use an immersion blender to puree the soup until smooth. If you prefer a chunkier texture, blend only half of the soup.

6. Stir in the shredded cheddar cheese until melted and fully incorporated.

7. Season with black pepper and paprika. Serve hot.

Nutrition (per serving):

- Calories: 200

- Protein: 12g

- Carbohydrates: 15g

- Fat: 10g

- Sodium: 240mg

- Potassium: 400mg

Spinach and Feta Wrap

Preparation Time: 10 minutes

Cooking Time: 5 minutes

Servings: 4

Ingredients:

- 4 whole wheat tortillas

- 2 cups fresh spinach leaves

- 1/2 cup crumbled feta cheese

- 1 small red bell pepper, thinly sliced

- 1 small cucumber, thinly sliced

- 2 tablespoons hummus

- 1 tablespoon olive oil

- 1/4 teaspoon black pepper

Directions:

1. Heat the olive oil in a skillet over medium heat. Add the red bell pepper and cook for 5 minutes until tender.

2. Spread a thin layer of hummus on each tortilla.

3. Layer the spinach leaves, cooked bell pepper, cucumber slices, and crumbled feta cheese on top of the hummus.

4. Sprinkle with black pepper.

5. Roll up the tortillas tightly and slice in half. Serve immediately.

Nutrition (per serving):

- Calories: 220

- Protein: 8g

- Carbohydrates: 26g

- Fat: 10g

- Sodium: 350mg

- Potassium: 300mg

Summer Squash Soup

Preparation Time: 10 minutes

Cooking Time: 25 minutes

Servings: 4

Ingredients:

- 4 cups summer squash, chopped

- 1 small onion, chopped

- 2 cloves garlic, minced

- 3 cups low-sodium vegetable broth

- 1 tablespoon olive oil

- 1/4 cup fresh basil leaves, chopped

- 1/4 teaspoon black pepper

- 1/4 teaspoon salt (optional)

Directions:

1. Heat the olive oil in a large pot over medium heat. Add the onion and garlic, sautéing until softened, about 5 minutes.

2. Add the chopped summer squash and cook for another 5 minutes, stirring occasionally.

3. Pour in the vegetable broth and bring the mixture to a boil. Reduce the heat and let it simmer for 15 minutes, until the squash is tender.

4. Use an immersion blender to puree the soup until smooth.

5. Stir in the chopped basil leaves and season with black pepper and salt to taste. Serve hot.

Nutrition (per serving):

- Calories: 100

- Protein: 2g

- Carbohydrates: 10g

- Fat: 5g

- Sodium: 150mg

- Potassium: 350mg

Berry Spinach Salad

Preparation Time: 10 minutes

Cooking Time: None

Servings: 4

Ingredients:

- 4 cups fresh spinach leaves

- 1 cup fresh strawberries, sliced

- 1/2 cup fresh blueberries

- 1/2 cup fresh raspberries

- 1/4 cup crumbled goat cheese

- 1/4 cup chopped walnuts

- 2 tablespoons balsamic vinegar

- 1 tablespoon olive oil

- 1 teaspoon honey

- 1/4 teaspoon black pepper

Directions:

1. In a large bowl, combine the spinach leaves, strawberries, blueberries, raspberries, crumbled goat cheese, and chopped walnuts.

2. In a small bowl, whisk together the balsamic vinegar, olive oil, honey, and black pepper.

3. Drizzle the dressing over the salad and toss gently to combine.

4. Serve immediately.

Nutrition (per serving):

- Calories: 200

- Protein: 5g

- Carbohydrates: 20g

- Fat: 12g

- Sodium: 100mg

- Potassium: 450mg

Chapter 4:

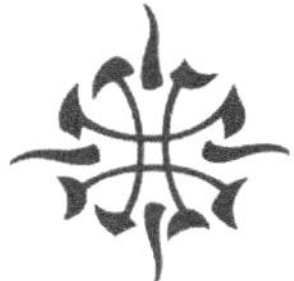

Baked Lemon Herb Chicken

Preparation Time: 10 minutes

Cooking Time: 35 minutes

Servings: 4

Ingredients:

- 4 boneless, skinless chicken breasts

- 2 tablespoons olive oil

- Juice of 2 lemons

- 2 cloves garlic, minced

- 1 teaspoon dried oregano

- 1 teaspoon dried thyme

- 1/2 teaspoon salt (optional)

- 1/4 teaspoon black pepper

- Lemon slices for garnish

- Fresh parsley for garnish

Directions:

1. Preheat your oven to 375°F (190°C).

2. In a small bowl, mix together the olive oil, lemon juice, garlic, oregano, thyme, salt, and black pepper.

3. Place the chicken breasts in a baking dish and pour the lemon herb mixture over them, making sure they are well coated.

4. Arrange lemon slices on top of the chicken breasts.

5. Bake in the preheated oven for 30-35 minutes, or until the chicken is cooked through and no longer pink in the center.

6. Garnish with fresh parsley and serve hot.

Nutrition (per serving):

- Calories: 220

- Protein: 28g

- Carbohydrates: 3g

- Fat: 10g

- Sodium: 220mg

- Potassium: 450mg

Grilled Salmon with Asparagus

Preparation Time: 10 minutes

Cooking Time: 15 minutes

Servings: 4

Ingredients:

- 4 salmon fillets

- 1 bunch asparagus, trimmed

- 2 tablespoons olive oil

- Juice of 1 lemon

- 2 cloves garlic, minced

- 1 teaspoon dried dill

- 1/2 teaspoon salt (optional)

- 1/4 teaspoon black pepper

- Lemon wedges for garnish

Directions:

1. Preheat the grill to medium-high heat.

2. In a small bowl, mix together the olive oil, lemon juice, garlic, dill, salt, and black pepper.

3. Brush the salmon fillets and asparagus with the olive oil mixture.

4. Grill the salmon fillets for about 5-7 minutes per side, or until the salmon is cooked through and flakes easily with a fork.

5. Grill the asparagus for about 5 minutes, turning occasionally, until tender.

6. Serve the grilled salmon with asparagus on the side, garnished with lemon wedges.

Nutrition (per serving):

- Calories: 350

- Protein: 30g

- Carbohydrates: 6g

- Fat: 22g

- Sodium: 180mg

- Potassium: 800mg

Turkey Meatloaf

Preparation Time: 15 minutes

Cooking Time: 60 minutes

Servings: 6

Ingredients:

- 1 1/2 pounds ground turkey

- 1 small onion, finely chopped

- 1 carrot, grated

- 1 celery stalk, finely chopped

- 1/2 cup whole wheat bread crumbs

- 1/4 cup low-fat milk

- 2 tablespoons ketchup (low-sodium)

- 1 tablespoon Worcestershire sauce

- 1 egg, beaten

- 2 cloves garlic, minced

- 1 teaspoon dried thyme

- 1/2 teaspoon salt (optional)

- 1/4 teaspoon black pepper

Directions:

1. Preheat your oven to 350°F (175°C).

2. In a large bowl, combine the ground turkey, onion, carrot, celery, bread crumbs, milk, ketchup, Worcestershire sauce, egg, garlic, thyme, salt, and black pepper. Mix until well combined.

3. Transfer the mixture to a loaf pan and press it down to form a loaf shape.

4. Bake in the preheated oven for 60 minutes, or until the meatloaf is cooked through and the internal temperature reaches 165°F (75°C).

5. Let the meatloaf rest for 10 minutes before slicing and serving.

Nutrition (per serving):

- Calories: 220

- Protein: 28g

- Carbohydrates: 10g

- Fat: 8g

- Sodium: 200mg

- Potassium: 500mg

Stuffed Portobello Mushrooms

Preparation Time: 15 minutes

Cooking Time: 25 minutes

Servings: 4

Ingredients:

- 4 large portobello mushrooms, stems removed

- 1 cup fresh spinach, chopped

- 1/2 cup cherry tomatoes, halved

- 1/4 cup red onion, finely chopped

- 1/4 cup feta cheese, crumbled

- 2 tablespoons olive oil

- 1 clove garlic, minced

- 1/2 teaspoon dried oregano

- 1/4 teaspoon black pepper

Directions:

1. Preheat your oven to 375°F (190°C).

2. In a skillet, heat 1 tablespoon of olive oil over medium heat. Add the garlic and onion, sautéing until softened, about 5 minutes.

3. Add the chopped spinach and cherry tomatoes to the skillet, cooking until the spinach is wilted, about 2-3 minutes.

4. Place the portobello mushrooms on a baking sheet. Brush the mushrooms with the remaining olive oil.

5. Spoon the spinach mixture evenly into each mushroom cap.

6. Sprinkle with crumbled feta cheese and dried oregano.

7. Bake in the preheated oven for 20-25 minutes, until the mushrooms are tender and the filling is heated through.

8. Serve hot, garnished with black pepper.

Nutrition (per serving):

- Calories: 180

- Protein: 5g

- Carbohydrates: 10g

- Fat: 14g

- Sodium: 200mg

- Potassium: 450mg

Roasted Garlic and Herb Pork Tenderloin

Preparation Time: 15 minutes

Cooking Time: 30 minutes

Servings: 4

Ingredients:

- 1 1/2 pounds pork tenderloin

- 4 cloves garlic, minced

- 2 tablespoons olive oil

- 1 tablespoon fresh rosemary, chopped

- 1 tablespoon fresh thyme, chopped

- Juice of 1 lemon

- 1/2 teaspoon salt (optional)

- 1/4 teaspoon black pepper

Directions:

1. Preheat your oven to 400°F (200°C).

2. In a small bowl, combine the minced garlic, olive oil, rosemary, thyme, lemon juice, salt, and black pepper.

3. Rub the garlic and herb mixture all over the pork tenderloin.

4. Place the pork tenderloin in a roasting pan and roast in the preheated oven for 25-30 minutes, or until the internal temperature reaches 145°F (63°C).

5. Let the pork rest for 10 minutes before slicing and serving.

Nutrition (per serving):

- Calories: 250

- Protein: 27g

- Carbohydrates: 2g

- Fat: 15g

- Sodium: 220mg

- Potassium: 500mg

Spaghetti Squash with Tomato Basil Sauce

Preparation Time: 15 minutes

Cooking Time: 40 minutes

Servings: 4

Ingredients:

- 1 large spaghetti squash

- 2 cups cherry tomatoes, halved

- 1/2 cup fresh basil leaves, chopped

- 1 small onion, chopped

- 2 cloves garlic, minced

- 2 tablespoons olive oil

- 1/4 teaspoon salt (optional)

- 1/4 teaspoon black pepper

- 1/4 cup grated Parmesan cheese (optional)

Directions:

1. Preheat your oven to 400°F (200°C). Cut the spaghetti squash in half lengthwise and remove the seeds.

2. Place the squash halves cut side down on a baking sheet and bake for 30-40 minutes, or until tender.

3. While the squash is baking, heat the olive oil in a skillet over medium heat. Add the onion and garlic, sautéing until softened, about 5 minutes.

4. Add the cherry tomatoes, salt, and black pepper, cooking for another 10 minutes, until the tomatoes are soft and the sauce is slightly thickened.

5. Remove the squash from the oven and use a fork to scrape out the strands into a bowl.

6. Toss the spaghetti squash with the tomato basil sauce and sprinkle with grated Parmesan cheese if desired. Serve hot.

Nutrition (per serving):

- Calories: 180

- Protein: 4g

- Carbohydrates: 18g

- Fat: 10g

- Sodium: 180mg

- Potassium: 600mg

Baked Tilapia with Lemon and Dill

Preparation Time: 10 minutes

Cooking Time: 20 minutes

Servings: 4

Ingredients:

- 4 tilapia fillets

- 2 tablespoons olive oil

- Juice of 1 lemon

- 1 tablespoon fresh dill, chopped

- 2 cloves garlic, minced

- 1/4 teaspoon salt (optional)

- 1/4 teaspoon black pepper

- Lemon slices for garnish

Directions:

1. Preheat your oven to 375°F (190°C).

2. In a small bowl, mix together the olive oil, lemon juice, dill, garlic, salt, and black pepper.

3. Place the tilapia fillets in a baking dish and brush the lemon dill mixture over them.

4. Bake in the preheated oven for 15-20 minutes, or until the fish is cooked through and flakes easily with a fork.

5. Garnish with lemon slices and serve hot.

Nutrition (per serving):

- Calories: 200

- Protein: 22g

- Carbohydrates: 2g

- Fat: 11g

- Sodium: 150mg

- Potassium: 450mg

Lentil and Vegetable Stew

Preparation Time: 15 minutes

Cooking Time: 40 minutes

Servings: 6

Ingredients:

- 1 cup dried lentils, rinsed

- 1 small onion, chopped

- 2 carrots, chopped

- 2 celery stalks, chopped

- 2 cloves garlic, minced

- 1 can (14.5 oz) diced tomatoes (no salt added)

- 4 cups low-sodium vegetable broth

- 1 tablespoon olive oil

- 1 teaspoon dried thyme

- 1 teaspoon dried oregano

- 1/2 teaspoon cumin

- 1/4 teaspoon black pepper

- 2 cups fresh spinach leaves

Directions:

1. Heat the olive oil in a large pot over medium heat. Add the onion, carrots, celery, and garlic, sautéing until softened, about 5 minutes.

2. Stir in the lentils, diced tomatoes, vegetable broth, thyme, oregano, cumin, and black pepper.

3. Bring the mixture to a boil, then reduce the heat and let it simmer for 30-35 minutes, or until the lentils are tender.

4. Stir in the fresh spinach leaves and cook for an additional 5 minutes, until the spinach is wilted.

5. Serve hot.

Nutrition (per serving):

- Calories: 250

- Protein: 12g

- Carbohydrates: 40g

- Fat: 5g

- Sodium: 150mg

- Potassium: 750mg

Preparation Time: 15 minutes

Cooking Time: 15 minutes

Servings: 4

Ingredients:

- 1 pound lean beef sirloin, thinly sliced

- 2 cups broccoli florets

- 1 red bell pepper, thinly sliced

- 1 small onion, sliced

- 2 cloves garlic, minced

- 2 tablespoons low-sodium soy sauce

- 1 tablespoon oyster sauce

- 1 tablespoon olive oil

- 1 teaspoon grated ginger

- 1/4 teaspoon black pepper

- Cooked brown rice for serving

Directions:

1. In a small bowl, mix together the soy sauce, oyster sauce, and grated ginger.

2. Heat the olive oil in a large skillet or wok over medium-high heat. Add the garlic and onion, sautéing for 2 minutes until fragrant.

3. Add the sliced beef to the skillet, cooking until browned, about 3-4 minutes.

4. Add the broccoli and red bell pepper, cooking for another 5-7 minutes until the vegetables are tender-crisp.

5. Pour the soy sauce mixture over the beef and vegetables, stirring to combine and heat through.

6. Season with black pepper and serve hot over cooked brown rice.

Nutrition (per serving):

- Calories: 300

- Protein: 25g

- Carbohydrates: 20g

- Fat: 12g

- Sodium: 400mg

- Potassium: 600mg

Zucchini Lasagna

Preparation Time: 20 minutes

Cooking Time: 45 minutes

Servings: 6

Ingredients:

- 3 large zucchinis, sliced lengthwise into thin strips

- 1 pound ground turkey

- 2 cups low-sodium marinara sauce

- 1 cup part-skim ricotta cheese

- 1 cup shredded mozzarella cheese

- 1/2 cup grated Parmesan cheese

- 1 egg

- 1 small onion, chopped

- 2 cloves garlic, minced

- 1 tablespoon olive oil

- 1 teaspoon dried oregano

- 1/2 teaspoon dried basil

- 1/4 teaspoon black pepper

Directions:

1. Preheat your oven to 375°F (190°C).

2. Heat the olive oil in a large skillet over medium heat. Add the onion and garlic, sautéing until softened, about 5 minutes.

3. Add the ground turkey, cooking until browned and no longer pink. Stir in the marinara sauce, oregano, basil, and black pepper. Simmer for 10 minutes.

4. In a bowl, mix together the ricotta cheese, egg, and 1/4 cup Parmesan cheese.

5. In a 9x13-inch baking dish, spread a thin layer of the meat sauce. Layer with zucchini slices, then spread some of the ricotta mixture over the zucchini. Repeat the layers until all ingredients are used, finishing with a layer of meat sauce.

6. Sprinkle the top with mozzarella cheese and the remaining Parmesan cheese.

7. Bake in the preheated oven for 35-45 minutes, until the cheese is bubbly and golden. Let rest for 10 minutes before slicing and serving.

Nutrition (per serving):

- Calories: 320

- Protein: 25g

- Carbohydrates: 10g

- Fat: 20g

- Sodium: 450mg

- Potassium: 750mg

Chicken and Vegetable Kabobs

Preparation Time: 20 minutes (plus 30 minutes marinating time)

Cooking Time: 15 minutes

Servings: 4

Ingredients:

- 1 pound boneless, skinless chicken breasts, cut into 1-inch cubes

- 1 red bell pepper, cut into 1-inch pieces

- 1 yellow bell pepper, cut into 1-inch pieces

- 1 red onion, cut into 1-inch pieces

- 1 zucchini, cut into 1/2-inch slices

- 1/4 cup olive oil

- Juice of 1 lemon

- 2 cloves garlic, minced

- 1 teaspoon dried oregano

- 1/2 teaspoon dried thyme

- 1/4 teaspoon salt (optional)

- 1/4 teaspoon black pepper

- Wooden or metal skewers

Directions:

1. In a bowl, whisk together the olive oil, lemon juice, garlic, oregano, thyme, salt, and black pepper.

2. Add the chicken cubes to the marinade, tossing to coat. Cover and refrigerate for at least 30 minutes.

3. Preheat the grill to medium-high heat.

4. Thread the chicken, bell peppers, onion, and zucchini onto skewers, alternating pieces.

5. Grill the kabobs for 10-15 minutes, turning occasionally, until the chicken is cooked through and the vegetables are tender.

6. Serve hot, garnished with additional lemon juice if desired.

Nutrition (per serving):

- Calories: 250

- Protein: 26g

- Carbohydrates: 8g

- Fat: 14g

- Sodium: 200mg

- Potassium: 600mg

Grilled Shrimp with Pineapple Salsa

Preparation Time: 20 minutes

Cooking Time: 10 minutes

Servings: 4

Ingredients:

- 1 pound large shrimp, peeled and deveined

- 1 tablespoon olive oil

- Juice of 1 lime

- 1/2 teaspoon chili powder

- 1/4 teaspoon salt (optional)

- 1/4 teaspoon black pepper

Pineapple Salsa:

- 1 cup fresh pineapple, diced

- 1/2 red bell pepper, diced

- 1/4 red onion, finely chopped

- 1 jalapeño, seeded and finely chopped

- 2 tablespoons fresh cilantro, chopped

- Juice of 1 lime

Directions:

1. In a bowl, toss the shrimp with olive oil, lime juice, chili powder, salt, and black pepper.

2. Preheat the grill to medium-high heat.

3. Thread the shrimp onto skewers and grill for 2-3 minutes per side, until pink and opaque.

4. While the shrimp is grilling, combine all the salsa ingredients in a bowl and mix well.

5. Serve the grilled shrimp with pineapple salsa on the side.

Nutrition (per serving):

- Calories: 200

- Protein: 22g

- Carbohydrates: 12g

- Fat: 8g

- Sodium: 300mg

- Potassium: 300mg

Eggplant Parmesan

Preparation Time: 20 minutes

Cooking Time: 45 minutes

Servings: 6

Ingredients:

- 2 large eggplants, sliced into 1/4-inch rounds

- 1 cup whole wheat breadcrumbs

- 1/2 cup grated Parmesan cheese

- 2 cups low-sodium marinara sauce

- 1 1/2 cups shredded part-skim mozzarella cheese

- 1/2 cup all-purpose flour

- 2 eggs, beaten

- 2 tablespoons olive oil

- 1 teaspoon dried basil

- 1 teaspoon dried oregano

- 1/4 teaspoon salt (optional)

- 1/4 teaspoon black pepper

Directions:

1. Preheat your oven to 375°F (190°C). Lightly grease a baking sheet with olive oil.

2. Set up a breading station with three shallow bowls: one with flour, one with beaten eggs, and one with a mixture of breadcrumbs, Parmesan cheese, basil, oregano, salt, and black pepper.

3. Dip each eggplant slice into the flour, then the egg, and finally the breadcrumb mixture, pressing lightly to adhere.

4. Place the breaded eggplant slices on the prepared baking sheet and bake for 20 minutes, flipping halfway through, until golden brown.

5. Spread 1/2 cup of marinara sauce in the bottom of a 9x13-inch baking dish. Arrange a layer of eggplant slices on top of the sauce. Spoon more marinara sauce over the eggplant and sprinkle with mozzarella cheese.

6. Repeat the layers, ending with marinara sauce and a final sprinkle of mozzarella and Parmesan cheese.

7. Bake for 25 minutes, until the cheese is bubbly and golden. Let the dish rest for 10 minutes before serving.

Nutrition (per serving):

- Calories: 280

- Protein: 15g

- Carbohydrates: 30g

- Fat: 12g

- Sodium: 450mg

- Potassium: 600mg

Turkey and Sweet Potato Casserole

Preparation Time: 20 minutes

Cooking Time: 45 minutes

Servings: 6

Ingredients:

- 1 pound ground turkey

- 2 large sweet potatoes, peeled and cubed

- 1 small onion, chopped

- 2 cloves garlic, minced

- 1 cup low-sodium chicken broth

- 1 cup frozen peas and carrots

- 1/2 cup shredded low-fat cheddar cheese

- 2 tablespoons olive oil

- 1 teaspoon dried thyme

- 1/2 teaspoon dried sage

- 1/4 teaspoon salt (optional)

- 1/4 teaspoon black pepper

Directions:

1. Preheat your oven to 375°F (190°C).

2. Place the sweet potato cubes in a large pot of boiling water and cook until tender, about 10-15 minutes. Drain and mash with a fork or potato masher.

3. While the sweet potatoes are cooking, heat 1 tablespoon of olive oil in a large skillet over medium heat. Add the onion and garlic, sautéing until softened, about 5 minutes.

4. Add the ground turkey to the skillet, cooking until browned and no longer pink. Stir in the thyme, sage, salt, and black pepper.

5. Add the chicken broth and frozen peas and carrots to the skillet, simmering for 5 minutes.

6. Spread the turkey mixture in the bottom of a 9x13-inch baking dish. Top with the mashed sweet potatoes, spreading evenly. Drizzle with the remaining olive oil and sprinkle with shredded cheddar cheese.

7. Bake in the preheated oven for 25-30 minutes, until the cheese is melted and bubbly. Let cool for 10 minutes before serving.

Nutrition (per serving):

- Calories: 320

- Protein: 22g

- Carbohydrates: 30g

- Fat: 14g

- Sodium: 250mg

- Potassium: 700mg

<table><tr><td align="center">*Lemon Rosemary Chicken Thighs*</td></tr></table>

Preparation Time: 15 minutes

Cooking Time: 40 minutes

Servings: 4

Ingredients:

- 8 bone-in, skin-on chicken thighs

- 3 tablespoons olive oil

- Juice and zest of 2 lemons

- 4 cloves garlic, minced

- 2 tablespoons fresh rosemary, chopped

- 1 teaspoon dried thyme

- 1/2 teaspoon salt (optional)

- 1/4 teaspoon black pepper

- Lemon wedges for garnish

Directions:

1. Preheat your oven to 400°F (200°C).

2. In a small bowl, mix together the olive oil, lemon juice, lemon zest, garlic, rosemary, thyme, salt, and black pepper.

3. Place the chicken thighs in a large baking dish. Pour the lemon rosemary mixture over the chicken, making sure each piece is well coated.

4. Bake in the preheated oven for 35-40 minutes, or until the chicken is cooked through and the skin is crispy and golden.

5. Garnish with lemon wedges and additional rosemary if desired. Serve hot.

Nutrition (per serving):

- Calories: 400

- Protein: 30g

- Carbohydrates: 4g

- Fat: 28g

- Sodium: 300mg

- Potassium: 400mg

Baked Cod with Herbs

Preparation Time: 10 minutes

Cooking Time: 20 minutes

Servings: 4

Ingredients:

- 4 cod fillets

- 2 tablespoons olive oil

- Juice of 1 lemon

- 2 cloves garlic, minced

- 2 tablespoons fresh parsley, chopped

- 1 teaspoon dried dill

- 1/2 teaspoon salt (optional)

- 1/4 teaspoon black pepper

- Lemon wedges for garnish

Directions:

1. Preheat your oven to 375°F (190°C).

2. In a small bowl, mix together the olive oil, lemon juice, garlic, parsley, dill, salt, and black pepper.

3. Place the cod fillets in a baking dish. Pour the herb mixture over the cod, making sure each fillet is well coated.

4. Bake in the preheated oven for 15-20 minutes, or until the fish is cooked through and flakes easily with a fork.

5. Garnish with lemon wedges and additional parsley if desired. Serve hot.

Nutrition (per serving):

- Calories: 200

- Protein: 25g

- Carbohydrates: 2g

- Fat: 10g

- Sodium: 180mg

- Potassium: 450mg

Cauliflower Mac and Cheese

Preparation Time: 15 minutes

Cooking Time: 25 minutes

Servings: 6

Ingredients:

- 1 large head cauliflower, cut into florets

- 2 tablespoons butter

- 2 tablespoons all-purpose flour

- 2 cups low-fat milk

- 1 cup shredded sharp cheddar cheese

- 1/2 cup grated Parmesan cheese

- 1/4 teaspoon garlic powder

- 1/4 teaspoon onion powder

- 1/4 teaspoon salt (optional)

- 1/4 teaspoon black pepper

- 1/4 cup whole wheat breadcrumbs

- 2 tablespoons chopped fresh parsley (optional)

Directions:

1. Preheat your oven to 375°F (190°C).

2. Steam the cauliflower florets until tender, about 10 minutes. Drain and set aside.

3. In a medium saucepan, melt the butter over medium heat. Whisk in the flour and cook for 1 minute, stirring constantly.

4. Gradually add the milk, continuing to whisk until the mixture is smooth and starts to thicken.

5. Remove the saucepan from heat and stir in the cheddar cheese, Parmesan cheese, garlic powder, onion powder, salt, and black pepper until the cheese is melted and the sauce is smooth.

6. In a large mixing bowl, combine the cooked cauliflower with the cheese sauce, tossing gently to coat.

7. Transfer the cauliflower mixture to a 9x13-inch baking dish. Sprinkle the breadcrumbs evenly over the top.

8. Bake in the preheated oven for 15 minutes, or until the top is golden brown and bubbly.

9. Garnish with chopped parsley if desired. Serve hot.

Nutrition (per serving):

- Calories: 220

- Protein: 10g

- Carbohydrates: 12g

- Fat: 14g

- Sodium: 300mg

- Potassium: 450mg

Chicken and Broccoli Alfredo

Preparation Time: 15 minutes

Cooking Time: 25 minutes

Servings: 4

Ingredients:

- 2 boneless, skinless chicken breasts, cut into bite-sized pieces

- 2 cups broccoli florets

- 8 ounces whole wheat fettuccine

- 1 cup low-fat milk

- 1/2 cup grated Parmesan cheese

- 2 cloves garlic, minced

- 2 tablespoons butter

- 1 tablespoon all-purpose flour

- 1/4 teaspoon salt (optional)

- 1/4 teaspoon black pepper

- 1 tablespoon olive oil

Directions:

1. Cook the fettuccine according to package instructions. Add the broccoli florets to the boiling pasta water during the last 3 minutes of cooking. Drain and set aside.

2. In a large skillet, heat the olive oil over medium-high heat. Add the chicken pieces and cook until browned and cooked through, about 5-7 minutes. Remove the chicken from the skillet and set aside.

3. In the same skillet, melt the butter over medium heat. Add the garlic and cook for 1 minute, until fragrant.

4. Whisk in the flour and cook for 1 minute, stirring constantly.

5. Gradually add the milk, whisking continuously until the mixture is smooth and starts to thicken.

6. Stir in the Parmesan cheese, salt, and black pepper, and continue to cook until the sauce is smooth and creamy.

7. Add the cooked chicken and broccoli to the skillet, tossing to coat with the Alfredo sauce.

8. Combine the sauce with the cooked fettuccine and broccoli, tossing to coat evenly. Serve hot.

Nutrition (per serving):

- Calories: 450

- Protein: 35g

- Carbohydrates: 40g

- Fat: 16g

- Sodium: 400mg

- Potassium: 650mg

<hr>

Herb-Crusted Pork Chops

Preparation Time: 15 minutes

Cooking Time: 25 minutes

Servings: 4

Ingredients:

- 4 bone-in pork chops

- 1/2 cup whole wheat breadcrumbs

- 1/4 cup grated Parmesan cheese

- 2 tablespoons fresh parsley, chopped

- 2 tablespoons fresh rosemary, chopped

- 2 tablespoons olive oil

- 2 cloves garlic, minced

- 1/2 teaspoon salt (optional)

- 1/4 teaspoon black pepper

- Lemon wedges for garnish

Directions:

1. Preheat your oven to 375°F (190°C).

2. In a shallow dish, combine the breadcrumbs, Parmesan cheese, parsley, rosemary, salt, and black pepper.

3. Brush the pork chops with olive oil and rub with minced garlic.

4. Press each pork chop into the breadcrumb mixture, coating both sides evenly.

5. Place the pork chops on a baking sheet and bake in the preheated oven for 20-25 minutes, or until the pork chops are cooked through and the crust is golden brown.

6. Garnish with lemon wedges and serve hot.

Nutrition (per serving):

- Calories: 350

- Protein: 30g

- Carbohydrates: 10g

- Fat: 20g

- Sodium: 300mg

- Potassium: 500mg

Vegetable Paella

Preparation Time: 20 minutes

Cooking Time: 40 minutes

Servings: 6

Ingredients:

- 1 1/2 cups Arborio rice

- 1 red bell pepper, diced

- 1 green bell pepper, diced

- 1 small onion, chopped

- 2 cloves garlic, minced

- 1 cup green beans, trimmed and cut into 1-inch pieces

- 1 cup cherry tomatoes, halved

- 1 cup frozen peas

- 4 cups low-sodium vegetable broth

- 1/4 cup olive oil

- 1 teaspoon smoked paprika

- 1/2 teaspoon saffron threads

- 1/2 teaspoon turmeric

- 1/4 teaspoon salt (optional)

- 1/4 teaspoon black pepper

- Fresh parsley, chopped (for garnish)

- Lemon wedges (for garnish)

Directions:

1. Heat the olive oil in a large, deep skillet or paella pan over medium heat. Add the onion and garlic, sautéing until softened, about 5 minutes.

2. Add the red and green bell peppers and green beans, cooking for another 5 minutes.

3. Stir in the Arborio rice, smoked paprika, saffron, turmeric, salt, and black pepper, cooking for 2 minutes to toast the rice slightly.

4. Add the vegetable broth, bringing the mixture to a simmer. Reduce the heat to low and cook, uncovered, for 20 minutes, stirring occasionally.

5. Stir in the cherry tomatoes and peas, cooking for an additional 10 minutes, or until the rice is tender and most of the liquid is absorbed.

6. Remove the pan from heat and let the paella rest for 5 minutes before serving.

7. Garnish with chopped parsley and lemon wedges. Serve hot.

Nutrition (per serving):

- Calories: 350

- Protein: 7g

- Carbohydrates: 60g

- Fat: 10g

- Sodium: 250mg

- Potassium: 550mg

Chapter 5:

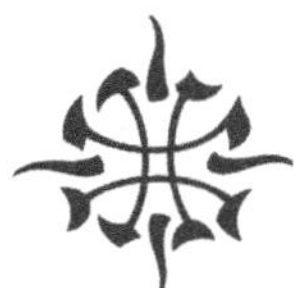

Roasted Chickpeas

Preparation Time: 5 minutes

Cooking Time: 40 minutes

Servings: 4

Ingredients:

- 2 cans (15 ounces each) chickpeas (garbanzo beans), drained and rinsed

- 2 tablespoons olive oil

- 1 teaspoon ground cumin

- 1 teaspoon paprika

- 1/2 teaspoon garlic powder

- 1/2 teaspoon salt (optional)

- 1/4 teaspoon black pepper

Directions:

1. Preheat your oven to 400°F (200°C). Line a baking sheet with parchment paper.

2. Pat the chickpeas dry with a clean kitchen towel or paper towels. Spread them out on the prepared baking sheet.

3. Drizzle the chickpeas with olive oil and sprinkle with cumin, paprika, garlic powder, salt, and black pepper. Toss to coat evenly.

4. Roast in the preheated oven for 30-40 minutes, stirring every 15 minutes, until the chickpeas are golden brown and crispy.

5. Remove from the oven and let cool slightly before serving.

Nutrition (per serving):

- Calories: 200

- Protein: 8g

- Carbohydrates: 25g

- Fat: 8g .

- Sodium: 200mg

- Potassium: 280mg

Low-Sodium Popcorn

Preparation Time: 5 minutes

Cooking Time: 5 minutes

Servings: 4

Ingredients:

- 1/2 cup popcorn kernels

- 2 tablespoons olive oil

- Salt-free seasoning blend (optional)

Directions:

1. Heat the olive oil in a large pot over medium-high heat. Add 3 popcorn kernels and cover the pot with a lid.

2. Once the test kernels pop, add the remaining popcorn kernels to the pot and cover again. Shake the pot gently to evenly distribute the kernels.

3. Continue cooking, shaking the pot occasionally, until the popping slows down to 2-3 seconds between pops. Remove from heat immediately.

4. Transfer the popcorn to a large bowl and season with salt-free seasoning blend if desired. Toss to coat evenly before serving.

Nutrition (per serving):

- Calories: 100

- Protein: 2g

- Carbohydrates: 15g

- Fat: 4g

- Sodium: 0mg

- Potassium: 50mg

Cucumber and Hummus Bites

Preparation Time: 10 minutes

Servings: 4

Ingredients:

- 1 large cucumber, sliced into rounds

- 1/2 cup hummus

- Fresh parsley leaves for garnish (optional)

Directions:

1. Arrange the cucumber slices on a serving platter.

2. Spoon a dollop of hummus onto each cucumber slice.

3. Garnish with fresh parsley leaves if desired. Serve immediately.

Nutrition (per serving):

- Calories: 60

- Protein: 3g

- Carbohydrates: 7g

- Fat: 3g

- Sodium: 120mg

- Potassium: 250mg

Sweet Potato Fries

Preparation Time: 10 minutes

Cooking Time: 25 minutes

Servings: 4

Ingredients:

- 2 large sweet potatoes, peeled and cut into fries

- 2 tablespoons olive oil

- 1 teaspoon paprika

- 1/2 teaspoon garlic powder

- 1/2 teaspoon onion powder

- 1/4 teaspoon salt (optional)

- 1/4 teaspoon black pepper

Directions:

1. Preheat your oven to 425°F (220°C). Line a baking sheet with parchment paper.

2. In a large bowl, toss the sweet potato fries with olive oil, paprika, garlic powder, onion powder, salt, and black pepper until evenly coated.

3. Spread the seasoned sweet potato fries in a single layer on the prepared baking sheet.

4. Bake in the preheated oven for 20-25 minutes, flipping halfway through, until the fries are golden brown and crispy.

5. Remove from the oven and let cool slightly before serving.

Nutrition (per serving):

- Calories: 150

- Protein: 2g

- Carbohydrates: 25g

- Fat: 6g

- Sodium: 120mg

- Potassium: 380mg

Baked Zucchini Chips

Preparation Time: 10 minutes

Cooking Time: 25 minutes

Servings: 4

Ingredients:

- 2 large zucchinis, thinly sliced into rounds

- 2 tablespoons olive oil

- 1/4 cup grated Parmesan cheese

- 1/2 teaspoon garlic powder

- 1/2 teaspoon dried oregano

- 1/4 teaspoon salt (optional)

- 1/4 teaspoon black pepper

Directions:

1. Preheat your oven to 425°F (220°C). Line a baking sheet with parchment paper.

2. In a large bowl, toss the zucchini slices with olive oil, Parmesan cheese, garlic powder, oregano, salt, and black pepper until evenly coated.

3. Arrange the seasoned zucchini slices in a single layer on the prepared baking sheet.

4. Bake in the preheated oven for 20-25 minutes, flipping halfway through, until the zucchini chips are golden brown and crispy.

5. Remove from the oven and let cool slightly before serving.

Nutrition (per serving):

- Calories: 80

- Protein: 3g

- Carbohydrates: 5g

- Fat: 6g

- Sodium: 150mg

- Potassium: 300mg

Apple Slices with Almond Butter

Preparation Time: 5 minutes

Servings: 4

Ingredients:

- 2 apples, cored and sliced

- 1/4 cup almond butter

Directions:

1. Arrange the apple slices on a serving plate.

2. Serve with almond butter for dipping or spreading.

Nutrition (per serving):

- Calories: 150

- Protein: 3g

- Carbohydrates: 15g

- Fat: 10g

- Sodium: 0mg

- Potassium: 200mg

Roasted Bell Peppers

Preparation Time: 10 minutes

Cooking Time: 20 minutes

Servings: 4

Ingredients:

- 2 bell peppers (any color), seeded and sliced

- 2 tablespoons olive oil

- 1 teaspoon dried thyme

- 1/2 teaspoon garlic powder

- 1/4 teaspoon salt (optional)

- 1/4 teaspoon black pepper

Directions:

1. Preheat your oven to 425°F (220°C). Line a baking sheet with parchment paper.

2. In a large bowl, toss the bell pepper slices with olive oil, thyme, garlic powder, salt, and black pepper until evenly coated.

3. Spread the seasoned bell pepper slices in a single layer on the prepared baking sheet.

4. Roast in the preheated oven for 15-20 minutes, stirring halfway through, until the peppers are tender and slightly charred.

5. Remove from the oven and let cool slightly before serving.

Nutrition (per serving):

- Calories: 60

- Protein: 1g

- Carbohydrates: 4g

- Fat: 5g

- Sodium: 75mg

- Potassium: 150mg

Carrot and Celery Sticks with Greek Yogurt Dip

Preparation Time: 10 minutes

Servings: 4

Ingredients:

- 2 carrots, peeled and cut into sticks

- 2 celery stalks, cut into sticks

- 1 cup Greek yogurt

- 1 tablespoon lemon juice

- 1 teaspoon dried dill

- 1/4 teaspoon garlic powder

- 1/4 teaspoon salt (optional)

- 1/4 teaspoon black pepper

Directions:

1. In a small bowl, mix together the Greek yogurt, lemon juice, dried dill, garlic powder, salt, and black pepper until well combined.

2. Arrange the carrot and celery sticks on a serving plate.

3. Serve with the Greek yogurt dip.

Nutrition (per serving):

- Calories: 50

- Protein: 4g

- Carbohydrates: 6g

- Fat: 1g

- Sodium: 100mg

- Potassium: 200mg

Preparation Time: 10 minutes

Marinating Time: 1 hour

Servings: 4

Ingredients:

- 1 cup mixed olives (such as Kalamata and green olives)

- 2 tablespoons olive oil

- 2 cloves garlic, minced

- 1 teaspoon lemon zest

- 1 teaspoon dried oregano

- 1/2 teaspoon red pepper flakes

- Fresh parsley for garnish (optional)

Directions:

1. In a bowl, combine the olives, olive oil, minced garlic, lemon zest, oregano, and red pepper flakes. Toss to coat the olives evenly.

2. Cover the bowl and let the olives marinate in the refrigerator for at least 1 hour, or overnight for best flavor.

3. Before serving, garnish with fresh parsley if desired. Serve chilled or at room temperature.

Nutrition (per serving):

- Calories: 100

- Protein: 1g

- Carbohydrates: 3g

- Fat: 10g

- Sodium: 300mg

- Potassium: 50mg

Kale Chips

Preparation Time: 10 minutes

Cooking Time: 15 minutes

Servings: 4

Ingredients:

- 1 bunch kale, stems removed and leaves torn into bite-sized pieces

- 2 tablespoons olive oil

- 1 tablespoon nutritional yeast (optional)

- 1/2 teaspoon garlic powder

- 1/4 teaspoon salt (optional)

- 1/4 teaspoon black pepper

Directions:

1. Preheat your oven to 350°F (175°C). Line a baking sheet with parchment paper.

2. In a large bowl, toss the kale leaves with olive oil, nutritional yeast (if using), garlic powder, salt, and black pepper until evenly coated.

3. Spread the seasoned kale leaves in a single layer on the prepared baking sheet.

4. Bake in the preheated oven for 12-15 minutes, or until the kale chips are crisp and slightly browned.

5. Remove from the oven and let cool slightly before serving.

Nutrition (per serving):

- Calories: 70

- Protein: 2g

- Carbohydrates: 4g

- Fat: 5g

- Sodium: 100mg

- Potassium: 250mg

Strawberry and Basil Salad

Preparation Time: 10 minutes

Servings: 4

Ingredients:

- 4 cups baby spinach or mixed greens

- 1 cup fresh strawberries, sliced

- 1/4 cup fresh basil leaves, torn

- 2 tablespoons balsamic vinegar

- 1 tablespoon olive oil

- 1 teaspoon honey

- Salt and black pepper to taste

- 2 tablespoons sliced almonds (optional)

Directions:

1. In a large bowl, combine the baby spinach, sliced strawberries, and torn basil leaves.

2. In a small bowl, whisk together the balsamic vinegar, olive oil, honey, salt, and black pepper to make the dressing.

3. Drizzle the dressing over the salad and toss gently to coat.

4. Sprinkle sliced almonds over the top if desired. Serve immediately.

Nutrition (per serving):

- Calories: 70

- Protein: 2g

- Carbohydrates: 8g

- Fat: 4g

- Sodium: 50mg

- Potassium: 300mg

Garlic Mashed Cauliflower

Preparation Time: 10 minutes

Cooking Time: 20 minutes

Servings: 4

Ingredients:

- 1 large head cauliflower, cut into florets

- 2 cloves garlic, minced

- 2 tablespoons unsalted butter

- 1/4 cup low-fat milk or unsweetened almond milk

- Salt and black pepper to taste

- Chopped fresh parsley for garnish (optional)

Directions:

1. Steam the cauliflower florets until tender, about 10 minutes. Drain well.

2. In a large pot, melt the butter over medium heat. Add the minced garlic and cook for 1-2 minutes, until fragrant.

3. Add the steamed cauliflower to the pot, along with the milk. Use a potato masher or immersion blender to mash the cauliflower until smooth.

4. Season with salt and black pepper to taste. Cook for an additional 5 minutes, stirring occasionally, until heated through.

5. Transfer the mashed cauliflower to a serving dish and garnish with chopped fresh parsley if desired. Serve hot.

Nutrition (per serving):

- Calories: 60

- Protein: 2g

- Carbohydrates: 7g

- Fat: 4g

- Sodium: 45mg

- Potassium: 380mg

Beet Chips

Preparation Time: 10 minutes

Cooking Time: 25 minutes

Servings: 4

Ingredients:

- 2 large beets, peeled and thinly sliced

- 2 tablespoons olive oil

- 1 teaspoon smoked paprika

- 1/2 teaspoon garlic powder

- 1/2 teaspoon salt (optional)

- 1/4 teaspoon black pepper

Directions:

1. Preheat your oven to 375°F (190°C). Line a baking sheet with parchment paper.

2. In a large bowl, toss the beet slices with olive oil, smoked paprika, garlic powder, salt, and black pepper until evenly coated.

3. Arrange the seasoned beet slices in a single layer on the prepared baking sheet.

4. Bake in the preheated oven for 20-25 minutes, flipping halfway through, until the beet chips are crisp and slightly browned.

5. Remove from the oven and let cool slightly before serving.

Nutrition (per serving):

- Calories: 80

- Protein: 2g

- Carbohydrates: 10g

- Fat: 4g

- Sodium: 150mg

- Potassium: 300mg

Cucumber Salad with Vinegar

Preparation Time: 10 minutes

Servings: 4

Ingredients:

- 2 cucumbers, thinly sliced

- 1/4 cup white vinegar

- 2 tablespoons olive oil

- 1 tablespoon honey

- 1 teaspoon dried dill

- 1/4 teaspoon salt (optional)

- 1/4 teaspoon black pepper

- Thinly sliced red onion for garnish (optional)

Directions:

1. In a large bowl, combine the cucumber slices, white vinegar, olive oil, honey, dried dill, salt, and black pepper. Toss to coat the cucumbers evenly.

2. Let the cucumber salad marinate in the refrigerator for at least 30 minutes before serving.

3. Garnish with thinly sliced red onion if desired. Serve chilled.

Nutrition (per serving):

- Calories: 70

- Protein: 1g

- Carbohydrates: 6g

- Fat: 5g

- Sodium: 75mg

- Potassium: 250mg

Roasted Butternut Squash

Preparation Time: 15 minutes

Cooking Time: 30 minutes

Servings: 4

Ingredients:

- 1 medium butternut squash, peeled, seeded, and diced

- 2 tablespoons olive oil

- 1 teaspoon dried thyme

- 1 teaspoon smoked paprika

- 1/2 teaspoon garlic powder

- 1/2 teaspoon salt (optional)

- 1/4 teaspoon black pepper

Directions:

1. Preheat your oven to 400°F (200°C). Line a baking sheet with parchment paper.

2. In a large bowl, toss the diced butternut squash with olive oil, dried thyme, smoked paprika, garlic powder, salt, and black pepper until evenly coated.

3. Spread the seasoned butternut squash in a single layer on the prepared baking sheet.

4. Roast in the preheated oven for 25-30 minutes, stirring halfway through, until the squash is tender and caramelized.

5. Remove from the oven and let cool slightly before serving.

Nutrition (per serving):

- Calories: 90

- Protein: 1g

- Carbohydrates: 12g

- Fat: 5g

- Sodium: 150mg

- Potassium: 400mg

Sautéed Green Beans with Almonds

Preparation Time: 10 minutes

Cooking Time: 10 minutes

Servings: 4

Ingredients:

- 1 pound green beans, trimmed

- 2 tablespoons olive oil

- 1/4 cup sliced almonds

- 2 cloves garlic, minced

- 1/2 teaspoon lemon zest

- 1/4 teaspoon salt (optional)

- 1/4 teaspoon black pepper

- Lemon wedges for serving

Directions:

1. Heat the olive oil in a large skillet over medium heat. Add the sliced almonds and toast until golden brown, about 2-3 minutes.

2. Add the minced garlic and lemon zest to the skillet, cooking for 1 minute until fragrant.

3. Add the green beans to the skillet, tossing to coat with the garlic and almonds. Cook for 5-7 minutes, stirring occasionally, until the green beans are crisp-tender.

4. Season with salt and black pepper to taste. Serve hot with lemon wedges on the side.

Nutrition (per serving):

- Calories: 120

- Protein: 3g

- Carbohydrates: 9g

- Fat: 9g

- Sodium: 75mg

- Potassium: 300mg

Bell Pepper Strips with Guacamole

Preparation Time: 10 minutes

Servings: 4

Ingredients:

- 2 bell peppers (any color), seeded and sliced into strips

- 1 ripe avocado

- 1 tablespoon lime juice

- 1/4 teaspoon garlic powder

- 1/4 teaspoon onion powder

- 1/4 teaspoon salt (optional)

- 1/4 teaspoon black pepper

- Fresh cilantro leaves for garnish (optional)

Directions:

1. Arrange the bell pepper strips on a serving plate.

2. In a small bowl, mash the avocado with lime juice, garlic powder, onion powder, salt, and black pepper until smooth.

3. Serve the bell pepper strips with the guacamole for dipping.

4. Garnish with fresh cilantro leaves if desired. Serve immediately.

Nutrition (per serving):

- Calories: 80

- Protein: 2g

- Carbohydrates: 6g

- Fat: 6g

- Sodium: 75mg

- Potassium: 300mg

Steamed Edamame

Preparation Time: 5 minutes

Cooking Time: 5 minutes

Servings: 4

Ingredients:

- 2 cups frozen edamame (unshelled)

- 1 tablespoon sea salt (optional)

- Lemon wedges for serving

Directions:

1. Bring a pot of water to a boil. Add the frozen edamame and salt (if using).

2. Cook for 5 minutes, or until the edamame pods are tender.

3. Drain the edamame and transfer to a serving bowl.

4. Serve with lemon wedges for squeezing over the edamame pods before eating.

Nutrition (per serving):

- Calories: 120

- Protein: 9g

- Carbohydrates: 8g

- Fat: 4g

- Sodium: 0mg

- Potassium: 400mg

Spinach and Feta Stuffed Mushrooms

Preparation Time: 15 minutes

Cooking Time: 20 minutes

Servings: 4

Ingredients:

- 16 large button mushrooms, stems removed and reserved

- 2 cups fresh spinach, chopped

- 1/2 cup crumbled feta cheese

- 2 cloves garlic, minced

- 2 tablespoons olive oil

- Salt and black pepper to taste

- Chopped fresh parsley for garnish (optional)

Directions:

1. Preheat your oven to 375°F (190°C). Line a baking sheet with parchment paper.

2. Finely chop the reserved mushroom stems.

3. In a skillet, heat olive oil over medium heat. Add the chopped mushroom stems and minced garlic, cooking until softened, about 3 minutes.

4. Add the chopped spinach to the skillet and cook until wilted, about 2 minutes.

5. Remove the skillet from heat and stir in the crumbled feta cheese. Season with salt and black pepper to taste.

6. Spoon the spinach and feta mixture into the hollowed-out mushroom caps, filling each one generously.

7. Place the stuffed mushrooms on the prepared baking sheet and bake in the preheated oven for 15-20 minutes, or until the mushrooms are tender and the filling is golden brown.

8. Garnish with chopped fresh parsley if desired. Serve hot.

Nutrition (per serving):

- Calories: 120

- Protein: 6g

- Carbohydrates: 6g

- Fat: 9g

- Sodium: 200mg

- Potassium: 400mg

<table><tr><td> ***Lemon Dill Carrot Sticks*** </td></tr></table>

Preparation Time: 10 minutes

Cooking Time: 5 minutes

Servings: 4

Ingredients:

- 4 large carrots, peeled and cut into sticks

- 1 tablespoon olive oil

- 1 tablespoon fresh dill, chopped

- 1 tablespoon lemon juice

- 1/4 teaspoon garlic powder

- 1/4 teaspoon salt (optional)

- 1/4 teaspoon black pepper

Directions:

1. Steam the carrot sticks until tender, about 5 minutes. Drain well.

2. In a large bowl, toss the steamed carrot sticks with olive oil, fresh dill, lemon juice, garlic powder, salt, and black pepper until evenly coated.

3. Serve hot or chilled, depending on preference.

Nutrition (per serving):

- Calories: 60

- Protein: 1g

- Carbohydrates: 7g

- Fat: 4g

- Sodium: 150mg

- Potassium: 250mg

Chapter 6:

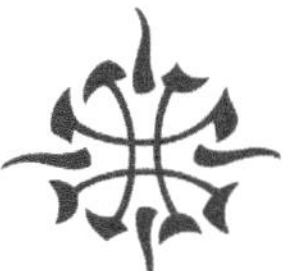

Mixed Berry Sorbet

Preparation Time: 10 minutes

Freezing Time: 4 hours

Servings: 4

Ingredients:

- 3 cups mixed berries (such as strawberries, blueberries, and raspberries), fresh or frozen

- 1/4 cup honey or maple syrup

- 1 tablespoon lemon juice

- Fresh mint leaves for garnish (optional)

Directions:

1. In a blender or food processor, combine the mixed berries, honey or maple syrup, and lemon juice.

2. Blend until smooth and well combined.

3. Pour the mixture into a shallow dish or baking pan.

4. Cover with plastic wrap and place in the freezer for at least 4 hours, or until firm.

5. Once the sorbet is frozen, use a fork to scrape the surface to create a flaky texture.

6. Serve in bowls or glasses, garnished with fresh mint leaves if desired.

Nutrition (per serving):

- Calories: 100

- Protein: 1g

- Carbohydrates: 25g

- Fat: 0g

- Sodium: 0mg

- Potassium: 150mg

Apple Crisp

Preparation Time: 15 minutes

Baking Time: 45 minutes

Servings: 4

Ingredients:

- 4 cups apples, peeled, cored, and sliced

- 1 tablespoon lemon juice

- 1/4 cup honey or maple syrup

- 1 teaspoon ground cinnamon

- 1/2 cup old-fashioned oats

- 1/4 cup almond flour

- 2 tablespoons coconut oil, melted

- 2 tablespoons chopped pecans or walnuts (optional)

Directions:

1. Preheat your oven to 350°F (175°C). Grease a baking dish with coconut oil.

2. In a large bowl, toss the sliced apples with lemon juice, honey or maple syrup, and ground cinnamon until well coated.

3. Transfer the apple mixture to the prepared baking dish, spreading it out evenly.

4. In the same bowl, combine the oats, almond flour, melted coconut oil, and chopped nuts (if using). Mix until crumbly.

5. Sprinkle the oat mixture over the top of the apples in the baking dish.

6. Bake in the preheated oven for 40-45 minutes, or until the topping is golden brown and the apples are tender.

7. Remove from the oven and let cool slightly before serving.

Nutrition (per serving):

- Calories: 250

- Protein: 3g

- Carbohydrates: 45g

- Fat: 8g

- Sodium: 0mg

- Potassium: 250mg

Preparation Time: 15 minutes

Baking Time: 25 minutes

Servings: 4

Ingredients:

- 1 cup almond flour

- 1/4 cup coconut flour

- 1/4 cup coconut oil, melted

- 1/4 cup honey or maple syrup

- Zest of 1 lemon

- 1/4 cup fresh lemon juice

- 2 eggs

- Powdered sugar for dusting (optional)

Directions:

1. Preheat your oven to 350°F (175°C). Grease a baking dish with coconut oil.

2. In a bowl, combine the almond flour, coconut flour, melted coconut oil, and honey or maple syrup. Mix until a dough forms.

3. Press the dough evenly into the bottom of the prepared baking dish.

4. Bake in the preheated oven for 10 minutes.

5. In another bowl, whisk together the lemon zest, lemon juice, and eggs until well combined.

6. Pour the lemon mixture over the partially baked crust.

7. Return to the oven and bake for an additional 15 minutes, or until the filling is set.

8. Let cool completely before cutting into squares. Dust with powdered sugar if desired.

Nutrition (per serving):

- Calories: 300

- Protein: 6g

- Carbohydrates: 25g

- Fat: 20g

- Sodium: 50mg

- Potassium: 150mg

Coconut Macaroons

Preparation Time: 10 minutes

Baking Time: 15 minutes

Servings: 4

Ingredients:

- 2 cups shredded coconut (unsweetened)

- 1/4 cup honey or maple syrup

- 2 egg whites

- 1 teaspoon vanilla extract

- Pinch of salt

Directions:

1. Preheat your oven to 350°F (175°C). Line a baking sheet with parchment paper.

2. In a bowl, combine the shredded coconut, honey or maple syrup, egg whites, vanilla extract, and salt. Mix until well combined.

3. Use a spoon or cookie scoop to portion out the mixture and shape into small mounds on the prepared baking sheet.

4. Bake in the preheated oven for 12-15 minutes, or until the coconut macaroons are golden brown around the edges.

5. Remove from the oven and let cool on the baking sheet for a few minutes before transferring to a wire rack to cool completely.

Nutrition (per serving):

- Calories: 200

- Protein: 3g

- Carbohydrates: 20g

- Fat: 12g

- Sodium: 70mg

- Potassium: 150mg

Chia Seed Pudding with Mango

Preparation Time: 5 minutes

Chilling Time: 4 hours or overnight

Servings: 4

Ingredients:

- 1/2 cup chia seeds

- 2 cups unsweetened almond milk or coconut milk

- 1 tablespoon honey or maple syrup (optional)

- 1 teaspoon vanilla extract

- 1 ripe mango, peeled and diced

- Fresh mint leaves for garnish (optional)

Directions:

1. In a bowl, whisk together the chia seeds, almond milk or coconut milk, honey or maple syrup (if using), and vanilla extract until well combined.

2. Cover the bowl and refrigerate for at least 4 hours or overnight, stirring occasionally, until the mixture thickens and sets into a pudding-like consistency.

3. To serve, divide the chia seed pudding into bowls or glasses. Top with diced mango and garnish with fresh mint leaves if desired.

Nutrition (per serving):

- Calories: 150

- Protein: 4g

- Carbohydrates: 20g

- Fat: 7g

- Sodium: 100mg

- Potassium: 180mg

Baked Apples with Cinnamon

Preparation Time: 10 minutes

Baking Time: 30 minutes

Servings: 4

Ingredients:

- 4 large apples, cored

- 2 tablespoons honey or maple syrup

- 1 tablespoon lemon juice

- 1 teaspoon ground cinnamon

- 1/4 teaspoon ground nutmeg

- 1/4 cup chopped walnuts or pecans (optional)

- Greek yogurt or vanilla ice cream for serving (optional)

Directions:

1. Preheat your oven to 375°F (190°C). Grease a baking dish with coconut oil.

2. Place the cored apples in the prepared baking dish.

3. In a small bowl, mix together the honey or maple syrup, lemon juice, cinnamon, and nutmeg.

4. Spoon the mixture into the center of each apple.

5. Bake in the preheated oven for 25-30 minutes, or until the apples are tender.

6. Remove from the oven and let cool slightly before serving.

7. Optional: Sprinkle chopped walnuts or pecans over the baked apples before serving. Serve with Greek yogurt or vanilla ice cream if desired.

Nutrition (per serving):

- Calories: 150

- Protein: 1g

- Carbohydrates: 30g

- Fat: 3g

- Sodium: 0mg

- Potassium: 200mg

Blueberry Lemon Popsicles

Preparation Time: 10 minutes

Freezing Time: 4 hours or overnight

Servings: 4

Ingredients:

- 2 cups fresh or frozen blueberries

- 1/4 cup honey or maple syrup

- 1 tablespoon fresh lemon juice

- Zest of 1 lemon

- 1 cup plain Greek yogurt

Directions:

1. In a blender, combine the blueberries, honey or maple syrup, lemon juice, and lemon zest. Blend until smooth.

2. In a separate bowl, mix the blueberry mixture with Greek yogurt until well combined.

3. Pour the mixture into popsicle molds.

4. Insert popsicle sticks into the molds and freeze for at least 4 hours or overnight until solid.

5. To unmold, run warm water over the outside of the molds for a few seconds and gently pull the popsicles out.

6. Serve immediately or store in the freezer in an airtight container.

Nutrition (per serving):

- Calories: 120

- Protein: 4g

- Carbohydrates: 20g

- Fat: 3g

- Sodium: 20mg

- Potassium: 150mg

Low-Sugar Banana Bread

Preparation Time: 15 minutes

Baking Time: 50 minutes

Servings: 8

Ingredients:

- 3 ripe bananas, mashed

- 1/4 cup unsweetened applesauce

- 1/4 cup coconut oil, melted

- 2 eggs

- 1 teaspoon vanilla extract

- 1 1/2 cups whole wheat flour

- 1 teaspoon baking powder

- 1/2 teaspoon baking soda

- 1/2 teaspoon ground cinnamon

- 1/4 teaspoon salt

- 1/4 cup chopped walnuts or pecans (optional)

Directions:

1. Preheat your oven to 350°F (175°C). Grease a loaf pan with coconut oil or line with parchment paper.

2. In a large bowl, mix together the mashed bananas, applesauce, melted coconut oil, eggs, and vanilla extract until well combined.

3. In a separate bowl, whisk together the whole wheat flour, baking powder, baking soda, cinnamon, and salt.

4. Gradually add the dry ingredients to the wet ingredients, stirring until just combined. Do not overmix.

5. Fold in the chopped walnuts or pecans if using.

6. Pour the batter into the prepared loaf pan and smooth the top with a spatula.

7. Bake in the preheated oven for 45-50 minutes, or until a toothpick inserted into the center comes out clean.

8. Remove from the oven and let cool in the pan for 10 minutes before transferring to a wire rack to cool completely.

Nutrition (per serving):

- Calories: 200

- Protein: 4g

- Carbohydrates: 25g

- Fat: 10g

- Sodium: 150mg

Raspberry Gelato

Preparation Time: 10 minutes

Chilling Time: 4 hours or overnight

Servings: 4

Ingredients:

- 2 cups fresh or frozen raspberries

- 1/4 cup honey or maple syrup

- 1 cup plain Greek yogurt

- 1 teaspoon vanilla extract

- Fresh raspberries for garnish (optional)

- Mint leaves for garnish (optional)

Directions:

1. In a blender, combine the raspberries, honey or maple syrup, Greek yogurt, and vanilla extract. Blend until smooth.

2. Pour the mixture into a shallow dish or baking pan.

3. Cover with plastic wrap and freeze for at least 4 hours or overnight, stirring occasionally, until firm.

4. Once the gelato is frozen, scoop into bowls or glasses. Garnish with fresh raspberries and mint leaves if desired.

Nutrition (per serving):

- Calories: 150

- Protein: 6g

- Carbohydrates: 25g

- Fat: 2g

- Sodium: 25mg

- Potassium: 150mg

Preparation Time: 15 minutes

Baking Time: 20 minutes

Servings: 4

Ingredients:

- 1 cup pumpkin puree

- 1/4 cup honey or maple syrup

- 2 eggs

- 1 teaspoon ground cinnamon

- 1/2 teaspoon ground nutmeg

- 1/4 teaspoon ground cloves

- 1/4 teaspoon ground ginger

- 1/4 teaspoon salt (optional)

- Whipped cream for serving (optional)

Directions:

1. Preheat your oven to 350°F (175°C). Grease a mini muffin tin with coconut oil or line with parchment paper.

2. In a bowl, whisk together the pumpkin puree, honey or maple syrup, eggs, cinnamon, nutmeg, cloves, ginger, and salt (if using) until smooth.

3. Spoon the pumpkin mixture into the prepared muffin tin, filling each cavity about three-quarters full.

4. Bake in the preheated oven for 18-20 minutes, or until set and lightly golden around the edges.

5. Remove from the oven and let cool in the muffin tin for 5 minutes before transferring to a wire rack to cool completely.

6. Serve pumpkin pie bites with whipped cream if desired.

Nutrition (per serving):

- Calories: 120

- Protein: 3g

- Carbohydrates: 15g

- Fat: 5g

- Sodium: 75mg

- Potassium: 200mg

Almond Butter Cookies

Preparation Time: 10 minutes

Baking Time: 12 minutes

Servings: 4

Ingredients:

- 1 cup almond flour

- 1/4 cup almond butter

- 1/4 cup honey or maple syrup

- 1 egg

- 1 teaspoon vanilla extract

- 1/4 teaspoon baking soda

- Pinch of salt

Directions:

1. Preheat your oven to 350°F (175°C). Line a baking sheet with parchment paper.

2. In a bowl, mix together the almond flour, almond butter, honey or maple syrup, egg, vanilla extract, baking soda, and salt until well combined.

3. Roll the dough into small balls and place them on the prepared baking sheet.

4. Use a fork to flatten each cookie slightly and create a crisscross pattern on top.

5. Bake in the preheated oven for 10-12 minutes, or until golden brown around the edges.

6. Remove from the oven and let cool on the baking sheet for 5 minutes before transferring to a wire rack to cool completely.

Nutrition (per serving):

- Calories: 200

- Protein: 6g

- Carbohydrates: 15g

- Fat: 15g

- Sodium: 75mg

- Potassium: 100mg

Pear and Ginger Compote

Preparation Time: 10 minutes

Cooking Time: 15 minutes

Servings: 4

Ingredients:

- 2 ripe pears, peeled, cored, and diced

- 2 tablespoons honey or maple syrup

- 1 tablespoon lemon juice

- 1 teaspoon grated fresh ginger

- 1/2 teaspoon ground cinnamon

- Pinch of salt (optional)

Directions:

1. In a saucepan, combine the diced pears, honey or maple syrup, lemon juice, grated ginger, ground cinnamon, and salt (if using).

2. Cook over medium heat, stirring occasionally, for 10-15 minutes, or until the pears are tender and the mixture has thickened.

3. Remove from heat and let cool slightly before serving.

4. Serve pear and ginger compote warm or chilled, as a topping for yogurt, oatmeal, pancakes, or ice cream.

Nutrition (per serving):

- Calories: 80

- Protein: 1g

- Carbohydrates: 20g

- Fat: 0g

- Sodium: 0mg

- Potassium: 100mg

Chocolate Avocado Mousse

Preparation Time: 10 minutes

Chilling Time: 1 hour

Servings: 4

Ingredients:

- 2 ripe avocados

- 1/4 cup cocoa powder

- 1/4 cup honey or maple syrup

- 1 teaspoon vanilla extract

- Pinch of salt

- Fresh berries for garnish (optional)

Directions:

1. In a blender or food processor, combine the ripe avocados, cocoa powder, honey or maple syrup, vanilla extract, and salt.

2. Blend until smooth and creamy, scraping down the sides of the blender as needed.

3. Transfer the mousse into serving dishes or glasses.

4. Cover and refrigerate for at least 1 hour to chill and set.

5. Garnish with fresh berries before serving if desired.

Nutrition (per serving):

- Calories: 200

- Protein: 3g

- Carbohydrates: 20g

- Fat: 15g

- Sodium: 5mg

- Potassium: 400mg

Strawberry Shortcake

Preparation Time: 20 minutes

Baking Time: 15 minutes

Servings: 4

Ingredients:

- 1 cup all-purpose flour

- 2 tablespoons sugar

- 1 1/2 teaspoons baking powder

- 1/4 teaspoon salt

- 1/4 cup cold unsalted butter, cut into small pieces

- 1/3 cup milk

- 1 teaspoon vanilla extract

- 1 cup sliced strawberries

- Whipped cream for serving

Directions:

1. Preheat your oven to 425°F (220°C). Line a baking sheet with parchment paper.

2. In a large bowl, whisk together the flour, sugar, baking powder, and salt.

3. Cut in the cold butter using a pastry blender or fork until the mixture resembles coarse crumbs.

4. Stir in the milk and vanilla extract until just combined.

5. Drop the dough by spoonfuls onto the prepared baking sheet, forming 4 shortcakes.

6. Bake in the preheated oven for 12-15 minutes, or until golden brown.

7. Remove from the oven and let cool on a wire rack.

8. To serve, split the shortcakes in half horizontally. Top each bottom half with sliced strawberries and whipped cream, then cover with the top halves.

Nutrition (per serving):

- Calories: 250

- Protein: 4g

- Carbohydrates: 35g

- Fat: 10g

- Sodium: 200mg

- Potassium: 150mg

Pineapple Upside-Down Cake

Preparation Time: 20 minutes

Baking Time: 35 minutes

Servings: 4

Ingredients:

- 1/4 cup unsalted butter

- 1/2 cup brown sugar

- 1 can pineapple rings, drained

- Maraschino cherries for garnish

- 1 cup all-purpose flour

- 3/4 cup sugar

- 1 teaspoon baking powder

- 1/4 teaspoon salt

- 1/2 cup milk

- 1/4 cup vegetable oil

- 1 egg

- 1 teaspoon vanilla extract

Directions:

1. Preheat your oven to 350°F (175°C). Grease a round cake pan.

2. In a small saucepan, melt the butter over medium heat. Stir in the brown sugar until dissolved.

3. Pour the butter and sugar mixture into the bottom of the greased cake pan.

4. Arrange the pineapple rings on top of the butter and sugar mixture, placing a cherry in the center of each pineapple ring.

5. In a large bowl, whisk together the flour, sugar, baking powder, and salt.

6. In a separate bowl, whisk together the milk, vegetable oil, egg, and vanilla extract.

7. Gradually add the wet ingredients to the dry ingredients, stirring until just combined.

8. Pour the batter over the pineapple and cherries in the cake pan.

9. Bake in the preheated oven for 30-35 minutes, or until a toothpick inserted into the center comes out clean.

10. Remove from the oven and let cool in the pan for 10 minutes before inverting onto a serving plate.

Nutrition (per serving):

- Calories: 400

- Protein: 4g

- Carbohydrates: 65g

- Fat: 15g

- Sodium: 300mg

- Potassium: 150mg

Preparation Time: 10 minutes

Baking Time: 20 minutes

Servings: 4

Ingredients:

- 4 ripe peaches, halved and pitted

- 2 tablespoons honey or maple syrup

- 1 teaspoon ground cinnamon

- Pinch of salt

- Greek yogurt or vanilla ice cream for serving

Directions:

1. Preheat your oven to 375°F (190°C). Line a baking sheet with parchment paper.

2. Place the peach halves cut side up on the prepared baking sheet.

3. Drizzle the honey or maple syrup over the peach halves.

4. Sprinkle with ground cinnamon and a pinch of salt.

5. Roast in the preheated oven for 15-20 minutes, or until the peaches are tender and caramelized.

6. Remove from the oven and let cool slightly before serving.

7. Serve roasted peaches with a dollop of Greek yogurt or a scoop of vanilla ice cream.

Nutrition (per serving):

- Calories: 100

- Protein: 1g

- Carbohydrates: 25g

- Fat: 0g

- Sodium: 0mg

- Potassium: 250mg

Vanilla Almond Milk Pudding

Preparation Time: 10 minutes

Chilling Time: 2 hours

Servings: 4

Ingredients:

- 2 cups unsweetened almond milk

- 1/4 cup honey or maple syrup

- 1/4 cup cornstarch

- 1 teaspoon vanilla extract

- Sliced almonds for garnish (optional)

Directions:

1. In a saucepan, whisk together the almond milk, honey or maple syrup, and cornstarch until smooth.

2. Place the saucepan over medium heat and cook, stirring constantly, until the mixture thickens, about 5-7 minutes.

3. Remove from heat and stir in the vanilla extract.

4. Pour the pudding into serving dishes or glasses.

5. Cover and refrigerate for at least 2 hours to chill and set.

6. Garnish with sliced almonds before serving if desired.

Nutrition (per serving):

- Calories: 100

- Protein: 1g

- Carbohydrates: 20g

- Fat: 2g

- Sodium: 100mg

- Potassium: 150mg

Cranberry Orange Scones

Preparation Time: 15 minutes

Baking Time: 15 minutes

Servings: 4

Ingredients:

- 2 cups all-purpose flour

- 1/4 cup sugar

- 1 tablespoon baking powder

- 1/2 teaspoon salt

- 1/2 cup cold unsalted butter, cubed

- 1/2 cup dried cranberries

- Zest of 1 orange

- 1/2 cup milk

- 1 egg, beaten

- Turbinado sugar for sprinkling (optional)

Directions:

1. Preheat your oven to 400°F (200°C). Line a baking sheet with parchment paper.

2. In a large bowl, whisk together the flour, sugar, baking powder, and salt.

3. Cut in the cold butter using a pastry blender or fork until the mixture resembles coarse crumbs.

4. Stir in the dried cranberries and orange zest.

5. In a separate bowl, whisk together the milk and beaten egg.

6. Gradually add the milk mixture to the flour mixture, stirring until a dough forms.

7. Turn the dough out onto a lightly floured surface and knead gently a few times until smooth.

8. Pat the dough into a circle about 1 inch thick. Cut into 8 wedges.

9. Place the scones on the prepared baking sheet. Sprinkle with turbinado sugar if desired.

10. Bake in the preheated oven for 12-15 minutes, or until golden brown.

11. Remove from the oven and let cool on a wire rack before serving.

Nutrition (per serving):

- Calories: 350

- Protein: 6g

- Carbohydrates: 45g

- Fat: 15g

- Sodium: 400mg

- Potassium: 150mg

Lime Sherbet

Preparation Time: 10 minutes

Chilling Time: 4 hours or overnight

Servings: 4

Ingredients:

- 1 cup freshly squeezed lime juice

- 1 cup sugar

- 2 cups cold water

- Zest of 2 limes

- Mint leaves for garnish (optional)

Directions:

1. In a large bowl, whisk together the lime juice, sugar, and cold water until the sugar is dissolved.

2. Stir in the lime zest.

3. Pour the mixture into a shallow dish or baking pan.

4. Cover with plastic wrap and freeze for at least 4 hours or overnight, stirring occasionally, until firm.

5. Once the sherbet is frozen, use a fork to scrape the surface to create a flaky texture.

6. Serve in bowls or glasses, garnished with mint leaves if desired.

Nutrition (per serving):

- Calories: 200

- Protein: 0g

- Carbohydrates: 50g

- Fat: 0g

- Sodium: 0mg

- Potassium: 50mg

Chocolate Covered Strawberries

Preparation Time: 15 minutes

Chilling Time: 30 minutes

Servings: 4

Ingredients:

- 1 cup semi-sweet chocolate chips

- 1 tablespoon coconut oil

- 12 large strawberries, washed and dried

- Assorted toppings (chopped nuts, shredded coconut, sprinkles) (optional)

Directions:

1. Line a baking sheet with parchment paper.

2. In a microwave-safe bowl, combine the chocolate chips and coconut oil.

3. Microwave in 30-second intervals, stirring between each interval, until the chocolate is melted and smooth.

4. Holding each strawberry by the stem, dip it into the melted chocolate, swirling to coat evenly.

5. Place the dipped strawberries on the prepared baking sheet.

6. Optional: Sprinkle with assorted toppings before the chocolate sets.

7. Place the baking sheet in the refrigerator for 30 minutes, or until the chocolate is set.

8. Serve chocolate covered strawberries as a decadent dessert or snack.

Nutrition (per serving):

- Calories: 200

- Protein: 2g

- Carbohydrates: 25g

- Fat: 12g

- Sodium: 0mg

- Potassium: 150mg

Chapter 7:

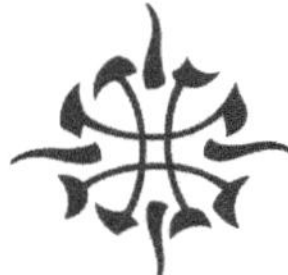

CONCLUSION

Maintaining a Balanced Diet with CKD

When managing chronic kidney disease (CKD), maintaining a balanced diet is crucial to supporting kidney function and overall health. Here are some key principles to keep in mind:

1. Monitor Protein Intake: Too much protein can strain the kidneys, so it's essential to consume the right amount. Work with a healthcare professional or dietitian to determine your individual protein needs and choose high-quality sources like lean meats, poultry, fish, eggs, dairy, and plant-based proteins such as beans, lentils, and tofu.

2. Control Phosphorus and Potassium: CKD can lead to imbalances in phosphorus and potassium levels in the blood. Limit foods high in phosphorus, such as dairy products, nuts, seeds, and processed foods. Similarly, manage potassium intake by avoiding high-potassium foods like bananas, oranges, tomatoes, and potatoes.

3. Watch Sodium Intake: Too much sodium can increase blood pressure and contribute to fluid retention. Limit processed foods, canned soups, salty snacks, and restaurant meals, and opt for fresh, whole foods seasoned with herbs and spices instead.

4. Choose Healthy Fats: Incorporate sources of healthy fats, such as olive oil, avocado, nuts, and seeds, into your diet while limiting saturated and trans fats found in fried foods, fatty meats, and packaged snacks.

5. Control Fluid Intake: Depending on your stage of CKD and individual health status, you may need to monitor fluid intake to prevent fluid buildup in the body. Limiting sodium can help reduce thirst and fluid retention, and tracking fluid intake throughout the day can help manage fluid balance.

6. Monitor Carbohydrates: Pay attention to carbohydrate intake and choose complex carbohydrates like whole grains, fruits, vegetables, and legumes over refined carbohydrates like white bread, sugary snacks, and desserts. Managing blood sugar levels is essential, especially for individuals with diabetes, which is a common complication of CKD.

7. Stay Hydrated: Drinking enough fluids is essential for kidney health, but individuals with CKD may need to limit their fluid intake depending on their condition. Work with your healthcare team to determine the right amount of fluids for you and choose hydrating options like water, herbal teas, and small portions of low-potassium fruits.

8. Consider Individual Needs: Every person with CKD is unique, so it's essential to tailor dietary recommendations to individual health status, stage of kidney disease, medications, and other factors. Regular monitoring and communication with healthcare providers and dietitians are key to ensuring a balanced and personalized diet plan.

Tips for Dining Out

Dining out can be enjoyable and convenient, but it can also present challenges for individuals with chronic kidney disease (CKD) who need to follow a specific diet plan. Here are some tips for navigating restaurant menus while managing CKD:

1. Plan Ahead: Before going to a restaurant, review the menu online if available. Look for dishes that are kidney-friendly and align with your dietary restrictions. Many restaurants offer nutrition information, which can help you make informed choices.

2. Customize Your Order: Don't hesitate to ask your server for modifications to meet your dietary needs. Request grilled or baked options instead of fried, ask for sauces and dressings on the side to control sodium and phosphorus, and substitute high-potassium sides with lower-potassium alternatives like steamed vegetables or a side salad.

3. Be Mindful of Portions: Restaurant portions are often larger than what you would eat at home, which can lead to overeating and consuming excess nutrients. Consider sharing an entree with a dining companion or asking for a half portion to manage portion sizes and avoid overindulging.

4. Choose Kidney-Friendly Options: Opt for dishes that feature lean protein sources like grilled chicken, fish, or tofu; whole grains like brown rice or quinoa; and plenty of vegetables. Avoid items that are high in sodium, phosphorus, and potassium, such as processed meats, creamy sauces, and heavily seasoned dishes.

5. Limit High-Phosphorus Additions: Be cautious of toppings and condiments that may be high in phosphorus, such as cheese, bacon, and pickles. Ask for these items to be served on the side or omitted from your meal to reduce phosphorus intake.

6. Drink Wisely: Be mindful of your beverage choices and opt for kidney-friendly options like water, herbal tea, or unsweetened iced tea. Limit or avoid sugary drinks, alcohol, and high-potassium beverages like orange juice and tomato juice.

7. Communicate with Your Server: If you have specific dietary restrictions or concerns, don't hesitate to communicate them to your server. They can help accommodate your needs and provide information about menu items and preparation methods.

8. Practice Portion Control: While it's tempting to indulge in appetizers, desserts, and extras, practice moderation to avoid consuming excess calories, sodium, and other nutrients. Consider sharing a dessert with your dining companions or saving half of your meal for later.

Staying hydrated is essential for kidney health, especially for individuals with chronic kidney disease (CKD). Proper hydration helps maintain kidney function, regulate body temperature, flush out toxins, and support overall health and well-being. Here are some tips for staying hydrated with CKD:

1. Monitor Fluid Intake: Depending on your stage of CKD and individual health status, you may need to monitor your fluid intake to prevent fluid overload and maintain fluid balance. Work with

Regular monitoring of your health is essential when managing chronic kidney disease (CKD) to track changes in kidney function, manage symptoms, and prevent complications. Here are some key aspects to monitor:

1. Blood Pressure: High blood pressure can worsen kidney damage, so it's crucial to monitor your blood pressure regularly. Aim for a target blood pressure of less than 130/80 mm Hg, as recommended by healthcare professionals.

2. Kidney Function Tests: Your healthcare provider may order blood tests to measure levels of creatinine, blood urea nitrogen (BUN), and glomerular filtration rate (GFR) to assess kidney function. These tests help determine your stage of CKD and guide treatment decisions.

179

3. Urine Tests: Urine tests, such as urinalysis and urine albumin-to-creatinine ratio (UACR), can provide information about kidney damage and protein leakage in the urine. Monitoring urine protein levels helps identify kidney disease progression and guide treatment strategies.

4. Electrolyte Levels: Monitoring electrolyte levels, including potassium, phosphorus, and calcium, is important for individuals with CKD to prevent imbalances that can lead to complications such as bone disease and heart problems.

5. Blood Sugar Levels: Individuals with CKD are at increased risk of developing diabetes, which can further damage the kidneys. Monitoring blood sugar levels and maintaining tight glycemic control is essential for preventing diabetes-related complications.

6. Symptoms and Complications: Pay attention to symptoms such as fatigue, swelling, changes in urine output, nausea, and difficulty breathing, as these may indicate worsening kidney function or complications requiring medical attention.

7. Medication Management: Keep track of your medications, including dosages and any side effects experienced. Discuss any concerns or changes in medication with your healthcare provider.

8. Lifestyle Factors: Monitor lifestyle factors such as diet, fluid intake, exercise, and stress levels, as these can impact kidney health and overall well-being. Making healthy choices and managing stress can help support kidney function and improve quality of life.